INTRODUCTION

The anatomical, physiological and biochemical adaptations that take place in women during the short span of human pregnancy are profound[1].

Pregnancy is a normal physiological phenomenon with many biochemical changes ranging from alterations in electrolyte concentrations to more complex changes in cortisol and Calcium metabolism. It is associated with normal physiological changes that assist in nurturing and survival of the fetus. Biochemical parameters reflect these adaptive changes and are clearly distinct from the non-pregnant state.

Preeclampsia is idiopathic multisystem disorder specific to human pregnancy. Hypertension is a universal problem; and it complicates at least 10% of all the pregnancies[2].

Preeclampsia is defined as the triad of hypertension, proteinuria and edema occurring after 20 weeks gestation in previously normotensive women[3]. It is transient but potentially dangerous complication of pregnancy. Preeclampsia is still one of the leading causes of maternal and fetal morbidity and mortality[4].

The pathophysiological mechanism is characterized by a failure of the trophoblastic invasion of the spiral arteries; leading to maladaptation of maternal spiral arterioles, which may be associated with an increased vascular resistance of the uterine artery and a decreased perfusion of the placenta[5].

However, the results from many clinical studies show the relationship between the aggravation of the hypertensive complications and the change in concentrations of various chemicals in mother's serum[6].

Interestingly, the significant reduction in serum Calcium and Magnesium are found in preeclamptic mothers. This result agrees with the physiological role of both Calcium and Magnesium in humans[7&8].

In this context, we have two major problems: delaying in early diagnosis and evaluating accurately the severity of this disease[9]. As the clinical process of Preeclampsia starts from the beginning of pregnancy, so it is important to diagnose it before progression of disease[10].

Due to this delay; many tests have attempted to establish the diagnosis of preeclampsia as early as possible, often even before the patient presents arterial hypertension[11]. Tests reported for the early diagnosis of preeclampsia are Doppler ultrasound assessment of maternal and fetal circulation[12-14], Uric acid concentration[15], Supine pressure test[16,17and18], Angiotensin test[19], Microalbuminuria[20], Plasma fibronectin concentration[21], Plasma antithrombin activity[22], Calciuria and other tests which are of debatable efficacy and practicality.

Renal function changes are seen in symptom free women in whom Preeclampsia will eventually develop. Several researchers evaluated the role of Calcium/Creatinine Ratio in urine for prediction of Preeclampsia in pregnancy[23-25].

Renal excretion of Calcium increases during normal pregnancy. Urinary Calcium excretion in normal pregnancy is 350-650 mg/day, compared with 100-250 mg/day in non pregnant women. Excretion usually increases during each trimester with maximum levels reached during third trimester[26]. In its clinical phase, preeclampsia is a hypocalciuria state[27]. In addition Calcium supplementation has shown promising results in patients at risk for preeclampsia[28]. Proteinuria has classically been an important sign in the diagnosis of preeclampsia.

There is hypocalciuria during normal pregnancy, while Preeclampsia is associated with hypocalciuria and low urinary Calcium creatinine ratio. This phenomenon occurs early enough and persists throughout gestation, so it is useful for early identification of patients at risk.

It is well known fact that electrolytes play an important role in aetiopathogenesis of hypertension[2].

Electrolytes like Calcium, Magnesium, Sodium and Potassium play an important role in preeclampsia as they contribute significantly in the functioning of the vascular smooth muscles[2]. Calcium plays a critical role in the function of vascular smooth muscles[2]. Alteration of plasma Calcium concentration leads to raised blood pressure. Magnesium act as co-factor for many enzymes (e.g. sodium potassium ATPase) and involved in peripheral vasodilatation[2,29and30]. Some studies shows that blood Calcium and Magnesium have a relaxant effect on the blood vessels of pregnant women[29,31].

On the basis of some studies claim that blood Calcium and Magnesium have a relaxant effect on the blood vessels of pregnant women[32].

Besides the serum Calcium and Magnesium, the hyperuricemia is believed to result from the decreased renal excretion that occurs as a consequence of the preeclampsia; also increased production may be secondary to tissue ischemia and oxidative stress. Soluble Uric acid impairs nitric oxide generation in endothelial cells. Hyperuricemia induces endothelial dysfunction and may induce hypertension and vascular diseases[5,6and33].

Therefore the modification of Calcium, Magnesium and Uric acid metabolism during pregnancy could be one of the potential causes of Preeclampsia.

The availability of highly sensitive and specific physiologic and biochemical markers would allow not only the detection of patients at risk but also permit a close surveillance, an exact diagnosis, timely intervention.

We are in acute need of a widely applicable and affordable test that could permit presymptomatic diagnosis in order to identify and monitor the mothers at risk and thus provide the best prenatal care for these women and their child. Such a test would also be of benefit to confirm a confounding clinical diagnosis and for future studies investigating prophylactic treatments.

Readily accessible routine and other Biochemical screening tests for Preeclampsia would ideally reduce the incidence of Maternal & Neonatal complications. It will also improve outcome of mother and fetus.

To be effective a screening test need to be sufficiently sensitive and specific and must provide an adequate positive predictive value[34].

Furthermore, when evaluating new screening strategies, not only sensitivity, specificity and predictive values should be taken into account, but also costs, patient's acceptability and quality control[35].

Preeclampsia in its severe form may be associated with cerebral or visual disturbances, oliguria, elevated serum creatinine and Uric acid along with the presence of epigastric pain. These changes when accompanied with convulsions or coma without pre-existing neurological disease like epilepsy, may lead to eclampsia.

Preeclampsia is a major cause for concern worldwide and there has been a constant search to find means for prediction and prevention. An availability of a good screening test would initiate more research in this direction and would ultimately pave the way for implementation of measures for primary prevention[36].

AIMS AND OBJECTIVES

As the pregnancy is a physiologic state, it is important to remember that pregnant women may often have some associated diseases, some of which may require biochemical investigations. The incidence of Preeclampsia is 10%; which also alter renal functions[2]. Now-a-days biochemical approach is implicated in order to prevent the complications in pregnancy and to improve the fetal outcome. There are various laboratory methods which can be useful in this regard. The aims and objectives of our study were:

- To determine the **predictive value of Calcium/Creatinine Ratio** in asymptomatic normotensive pregnant women in second trimester.

- The aim of this study was to measure S**erum levels of Calcium, Magnesium and Uric acid in preeclamptic women** and to compare those with normal pregnant women in third trimester.

- To develop a predictive model for Preeclampsia and subgroups at increased risk in whom prior therapy might be indicated to **prevent maternal and perinatal morbidity and mortality**.

- To introduce **Calcium/Creatinine Ratio in spot urine test** as a routine & economic **screening test for ANC profile**.

MATERIAL & METHODS

The study was conducted in *the Department of **Biochemistry** in collaboration with Department of **Obstetrics and Gynecology***, *Sri Aurobindo Medical College & Post Graduate Institute, Indore* during the period **January 2012 to January 2013**. The study protocol was approved by the institutional ethical committee and written informed consent was obtained from the subjects under study.

* SAMPLE SIZE: -

In the present study, the data have been collected from **100** asymptomatic, normotensive pregnant women between 20-28 weeks gestation, **100** pregnant women with diagnosis of Preeclampsia in the third trimester and **100** normal, age matched, healthy pregnant women in the third trimester that came to the Department of Obstetrics and Gynecology. The age of cases and control varied from 20 to 35 years with singleton pregnancy.

Subjects were divided into three groups:

Group–I: 100 asymptomatic, normotensive pregnant women between 20-28 weeks gestation (**For estimation of Urinary Calcium/Creatinine Ratio**). Out of 100 women, who were followed from 20-28 weeks of gestation till delivery, **Group-B** developed Preeclampsia whereas **Group-A** remained normotensive.

Group-II: 100 pregnant women with diagnosis of Preeclampsia in the third trimester (**For estimation of Serum Calcium, Serum Magnesium and Serum Uric acid**).

Group-III: 100 normal, age matched, healthy pregnant women in the third trimester i.e. **Control group for Group-II**.

* INCLUSION CRITERIA: -

- Asymptomatic pregnant women with gestational age 20-28 weeks of pregnancy with Blood pressure less than 130/80 mm Hg & no traces of Protein in urine (**For estimation of Urinary Calcium and Creatinine Ratio**).

- Mild Preeclamptic women with gestational age more than 28 weeks of pregnancy who had Proteinuria +1 or +2 detected by *Dip-stick Urine Analysis* method with Base-line Blood pressure more than or equal to 140/90 mm of Hg and had pitting Edema over feet (**For estimation of – Serum Calcium, Serum Magnesium and Serum Uric acid**).

- Asymptomatic pregnant women with gestational age more than 28 weeks of pregnancy with Blood pressure less than 130/80 mm Hg & no traces of Protein in urine (**For estimation of Serum Calcium, Serum Magnesium and Serum Uric acid**).

EXCLUSION CRITERIA:-

- Women with past history of Preeclampsia/Eclampsia.

- Women with the history of Diabetes mellitus.

- Women with the history of Chronic hypertension.

- Women with the history of Renal disease.

- Women with the history of any other Chronic illness.

- Women with Multiple pregnancies.

- Women under treatment of Anti-epileptic Drugs.

After taking written consent from the subjects, under all aseptic precautions, 3ml venous blood was collected in Vacutainer, allowed to clot and then immediately sent to the biochemistry lab. Where the samples were centrifuged at 4000rpm **x** for 10 minutes, then serum was separated and analyzed for the following tests:

1. Serum Calcium was estimated by **Arsenazo III method** (colorimetric) in *ERBA CHEM-5* (Enzymatic kit method).

2. Serum Uric acid by **Uricase method** in *ERBA CHEM-5* (Enzymatic kit method).

3. Serum Magnesium by **Calmagite method** in *ERBA CHEM-5*.

4. Blood Glucose by **Glucose Oxidase and Peroxidase method** in *ERBA CHEM-5*.

Spot urine sample of the subjects were also collected and be assessed in *Biochemistry lab* for the following tests:

1. Urine Calcium: Estimated by commercially available *standard enzymatic kits* with **VITROS 5,1 FS** (dry chemistry analyzer).

2. Urine Creatinine: Estimated by commercially available *standard enzymatic kits* with **VITROS 5,1 FS** (dry chemistry analyzer).

3. Urinary Protein: Estimated by **Dip-stick method**.

   Pre-test and post-test counseling was given to subjects.

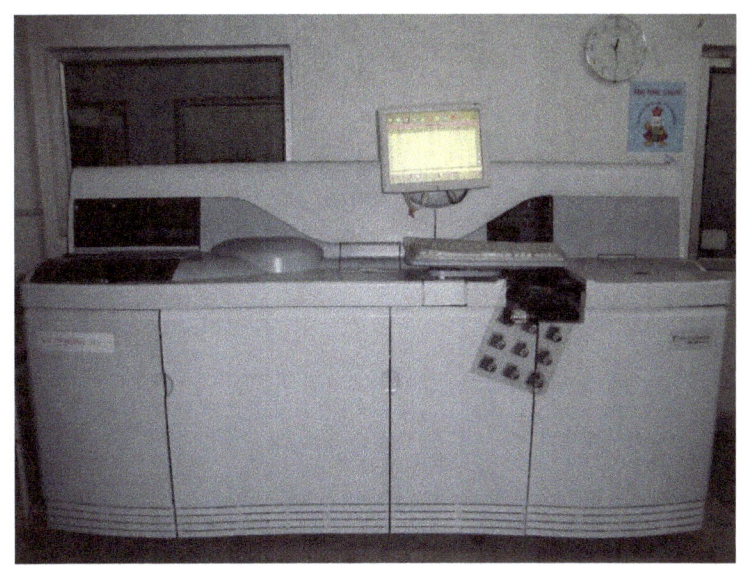

FIGURE 1: VITROS 5,1 FS

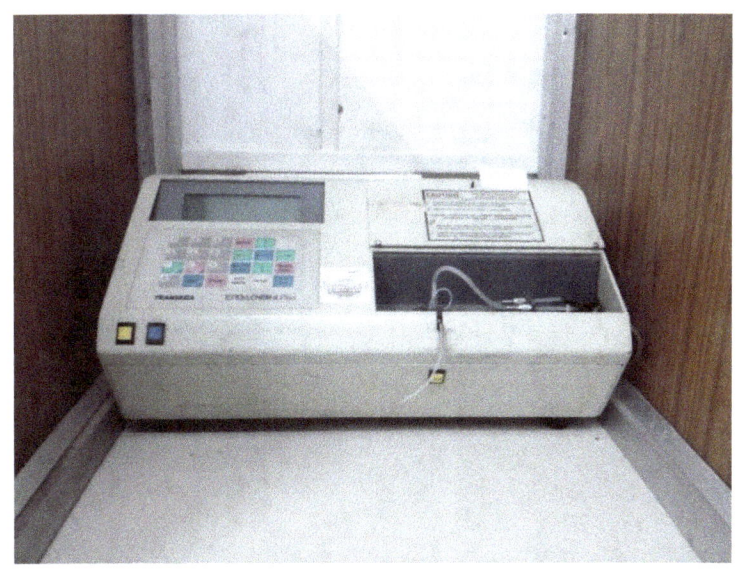

FIGURE 2: ERBA CHEM-5

METHODS

ESTIMATION OF SERUM GLUCOSE:

Blood Glucose by **Glucose Oxidase and Peroxidase method** in *ERBA CHEM-5.*

Principle:

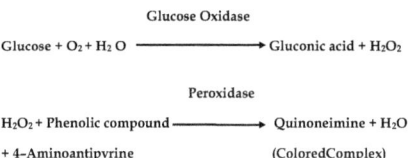

$$\text{Glucose} + O_2 + H_2O \xrightarrow{\text{Glucose Oxidase}} \text{Gluconic acid} + H_2O_2$$

$$H_2O_2 + \text{Phenolic compound} + \text{4-Aminoantipyrine} \xrightarrow{\text{Peroxidase}} \text{Quinoneimine} + H_2O \quad \text{(ColoredComplex)}$$

The intensity of colored complex produced is directly proportional to the concentration of glucose content and is measured at 505 nm (500-530 nm) on green filter.

Reagents:

1. Glucose (Enzyme, Chromogen buffer).

2. Glucose standard : 100 mg/dL

TABLE 1: Procedure

MODE	END POINT
Wavelength	505 nm (490-550nm)
Flow-cell temperature	37 ^{0}C
Optical path length	1 cm
Blanking	Reagent Blank
Sample volume	10 µL
Working Reagent volume	1000 µL
Incubation time	10 min. at 37 ^{0}C/30 min
Concentration of standard	100 mg/dL
Stability of color	1 hour
Permissible Reagent Blank absorbance	<0.2 AU
Linearity	Up to 500 mg/dL
Units	mg/dL

TABLE 2: Take three test tubes. Mark them as **T**-test, **S**-standard and **B**-Blank

Pipette into tube marked	Blank	Standard	Test
Serum/Plasma	-	-	10 µL
Reagent	-	10 µL	-
Working Glucose Reagent	1000 µL	1000 µL	1000 µL

- Calculate result as per given calculation formula.

Calculation:

$$\text{Serum/Plasma Glucose (mg/dL)} = \frac{\text{Absorbance of Test}}{\text{Absorbance of Standard}} \times 100$$

Normal Range:

    Fasting   : 70-110 mg/dL

    Postprandial   : <140 mg/dL

ESTIMATION OF SERUM CALCIUM[60]:

Serum Calcium was estimated by **Arsenazo III method** (colorimetric) by *ERBA CHEM-5* (Enzymatic kit method).

Principle:

Arsenazo III specifically binds to Calcium forming a colored complex which can be measured at 650nm.

Ca^{++} + Arsenazo III   ⟶   **Colored complex**

The amount of Calcium present in the sample is directly proportional to the intensity of the colored complex formed.

Concentration of working solution:

Mono-reagent:

Arsenazo III	-	200 µmol/L
MES pH 6.5	-	100 mmol/L
Standard	-	10 mg/dL

Sample material:

- **Serum**

- **Heparinized plasma**

- **Urine**: Diluted 1/3 with distilled water: acidified to pH 3-4 with N/10 HCl (consider dilution for calculation).

TABLE 3: Assay Procedure

Wavelength :	630		
Temperature :	25⁰ C - 37⁰C		
Read against reagent blank:	**Blank**	**Standard**	**Sample**
Reagent	1000 µL	1000 µL	1000 µL
Distilled water	10 µL	-	-
Standard	-	10 µL	-
Sample	-	-	10 µL

Mix and measure absorbance of the Sample A $_{(S)}$ and the standard A $_{(std)}$ against the absorbance of reagent blank A $_{(bl)}$ within 3 and 20 min.

$A_{(S)}$ = $A_{(S)}$ - $A_{(bl)}$

$A_{(STD)}$ = $A_{(Std)}$ - $A_{(bl)}$

Calculation:

$$\text{Concentration of sample} = \frac{\text{Absorbance of Sample}}{\text{Absorbance of Standard}} \times 10$$

(mg/dL)

Linearity:

Up to 16 mg/dL (4 mmol/L)

Normal Range: 8.10 – 10.4 mg/dL

ESTIMATION OF SERUM MAGNESIUM:

Serum Magnesium is estimated by **Calmagite method** *in ERBA CHEM-5.*

Principle:

Magnesium combines with Calmagite in an alkaline medium to from a red colored complex. Interference of Calcium and proteins is eliminated by the addition of specific chelating agents and detergents. Intensity of the color formed is directly proportional to the amount of Magnesium present in sample.

Alkaline Medium

Magnesium + Calmagite ⟶ Red colored complex

Magnesium kit:

Contents are:

     L1   :   Buffer Reagent

     L2   :   Color Reagent

     S   :   Magnesium Standard (2.0 mEq/L)

Procedure:

Wavelength/Filter	:	510 nm (Green)
Temperature	:	Room Temperature
Light path	:	1 cm.

TABLE 4: Pipette into clean dry test tubes labeled as Blank (**B**), Standard (**S**), and Test (**T**)

Addition Sequence	B (ml)	S (ml)	T (ml)
Buffer Reagent (L1)	0.5	0.5	0.5
Color Reagent (L2)	0.5	0.5	0.5
Distilled water	0.01	-	-
Magnesium Standard (S)	-	0.01	-
Sample	-	-	0.01

- Mix well and incubate at Room Temperature (25⁰C) for 5 min. Measure the absorbance of the Standard (Abs. S), and Test Sample (Abs. T) against the Blank, within 30 Min.

Calculation:

$$\text{Magnesium in mEq/L} = \frac{\text{Absorbance of Sample}}{\text{Absorbance of Standard}} \times 2$$

Linearity:

This procedure is linear up to 10mEq/L

Normal value: Serum Magnesium – 1.3 to 2.5mEq/L

ESTIMATION OF SERUM URIC ACID:

Serum Uric acid is estimated by **Uricase method** in *ERBA CHEM-5* (Enzymatic kit method).

Principle:

Uricase converts Uric acid into allantoin and hydrogen peroxide. In presence of peroxidase, hydrogen peroxide oxidatively couples with phenolic chromogens to from a red colored compound, which has maximum absorbance at 510 nm (500-530nm); the concentration of the red colored compound is proportional to the amount of Uric acid in specimen.

$$\text{Uric acid} + H_2O \xrightarrow{\text{Uricase}} \text{Allantoin} + H_2O_2$$

$$H_2O_2 + \text{Phenolic chromogen} \xrightarrow{\text{Peroxidase}} \text{Red color compound} + H_2O$$

Uric acid kit:

Components   **Concentration**

- Buffer, pH 7.8   :   > 150 mmol/L

- Peroxidase   :   > 100 IU/I

- Uricase   :   > 100 IU/I

- Ascorbate oxidase   :   > 100 IU/I

- Chromogen   :   1.0 mmol/L

- Activator & Stabilizer

TABLE 5: Procedure

Reaction type	End-Point
Reaction time	5 min at 37°C
Wave length (nm)	510 nm (500-530)
Zero setting with	Reagent Blank
Blank absorbance limit	<0.300 Abs
Sample	0.025 ml (25 µL)
Reagents volume	1.0 ml
Standard concentration	6 mg/dL
Linearity	25 mg/dL

Calculation:

$$\text{Concentration of sample (mg \%)} = \frac{\text{Absorbance of Sample}}{\text{Absorbance of Standard}} \times 6$$

Normal value:

Men: 3.4-7.0 mg/dL   &   **Wome**n: 2.4 – 5.7 mg/dL

ESTIMATION OF URINARY PROTEIN (BY URISTIX):

Procedure:

1. Dip reagent end of strip in fresh, well mixed, uncentrifuged urine and remove immediately.

2. While removing run the edge of the strip against the rim of the container to remove excess urine.

3. Compare reagent side of test areas with corresponding color charts at the times specified which shows quantitative values mentioned below:

+1   :   30 mg/dL

+2   :   100 mg/ dL

+3   :   300 mg/ dL

+4   :   Over 2000 mg/dL

ESTIMATION OF URINE CREATININE:

Urine Creatinine is estimated with commercially available standard enzymatic kits by **VITROS 5,1 FS** (Dry chemistry analyzer)

Principle:

The VITROS CREA slide is a multilayered, element coated on a polyester support. A drop of patient sample is deposited on the slide and is evenly distributed by the spreading layer to the underlying layers. Creatinine diffuses to the reagent layer, where it is hydrolyzed to creatine in the rate-determining step. The creatine is converted to sarcosine and urea by creatine amidinohydrolase. The sarcosine, in the presence of sarcosine oxidase, is oxidized to glycine, formaldehyde, and hydrogen peroxide. The final reaction involves the peroxidase catalyzed oxidation of a leuco dye to produce a colored product.

Following addition of the sample, the slide is incubated. During the initial reaction phase, endogenous creatine in the sample is oxidized. The resulting change in reflection density is measured at 2 time points. The difference in reflection density is proportional to the concentration of Creatinine present in the sample.

TABLE 6: Test type and Conditions

Test Type	VITROS System	Approximate Incubation Time	Temperature	Wave length	Reaction Sample Volume
Two-point rate	5,1 FS	5.0 minutes	37^0C (98.6^0F)	670 nm	6 µL

Reaction Scheme:

$$\text{Creatinine} + H_2O \xrightarrow{\text{Creatinine amidohydrolase}} \text{Creatine}$$

$$\text{Creatine} + H_2O \xrightarrow{\text{Creatine amidinohydrolase}} \text{Sarcosine} + \text{Urea}$$

$$\text{Sarcosine} + O_2 + H_2O \xrightarrow{\text{Sarcosine oxidase}} \text{Glycine} + \text{Formaldehyde} + H_2O_2$$

$$H_2O_2 + \text{Leuco dye} \xrightarrow{\text{Peroxidase}} \text{Dye} + 2H_2O$$

Reagents:

Slide Ingredients: Reactive Ingredients per cm^2

- Creatinine amidohydrolase (Flavobacterium sp. E.C.3.5.2.10) 0.20 U

- Creatine amidinohydrolase (Flavobacterium sp. E.C.3.5.3.3)4.7 U

- Sarcosine oxidase (Bacillus sp. E.C.1.5.3.1) 0.55 U

- Peroxidase (Horseradish root, E.C.1.11.1.7) 1.6 U

- 2-(3,5–dimethoxy–4-hydroxyphenyl)–4,5-bis(4-imethylaminophenyl) imidazole (leuco dye) 32 µg

Other Ingredients:

Pigment, Binders, Surfactants, Stabilizer, Scavenger, Chelator, Buffer, Dye solubilizer and Cross-linking agent.

Reagent's preparation:

IMPORTANT:

The slide cartridge must reach room temperature, 18-28⁰C (64-82 ⁰F), before it is unwrapped and loaded into the slide supply.

1. Remove the slide cartridges from storage.

2. Warm the wrapped cartridge at room temperature for 30 minutes when taken from the refrigerator or 60 minutes from the freezer.

3. Unwrap and load the cartridge into the slide supply.

Specimen Pre-treatment:

Urine: Predilution

Importance:

Using **VITROS 5,1 FS** Chemistry System in On-Analyzer Dilution Mode in which machine automatically mix 1 part of sample with 20 parts of reagent-grade water, analyze and multiply the result by 21 to obtain the Creatinine concentration in the original urine sample.

Measuring (Reportable or Dynamic) Range (mg/dL):

     Serum   -   0.05-14.0

     Urine   -   1.2-346.5

ESTIMATION OF URINE CALCIUM:

Urine Calcium is estimated with commercially available standard enzymatic kits by **VITROS 5,1 FS** (Dry chemistry analyzer)

Principle:

The **VITROS** Calcium slide is multilayered, analytical element coated on a polyester support. A drop of patient sample is deposited on the slide and is evenly distributed by the spreading layer to the underlying layers. The bound Calcium is dissociated from binding proteins, allowing the Calcium to penetrate through the spreading layer into the underlying reagent layer. There, the Calcium forms a complex with Arsenazo III dye, causing a shift in the absorption maximum. After incubation, the reflection density of the colored complex is measured Spectrophotometrically. The amount of colored complex formed is proportional to the Calcium concentration in the sample.

$$Ca^{++} + \text{Arsenazo III} \longrightarrow \text{Colored complex}$$

Slide Ingredients: Reactive Ingredients per cm^2

- Arsenazo III dye 60µg

 Other Ingredients:

Pigment, Binders, Surfactants, Buffer, Mordant and Cross-linking agent.

Regent's preparation:

IMPORTANT:

The slide cartridge must reach room temperature, 18-28^{0}C (64-82 ^{0}F), before it is unwrapped and loaded into the slide supply.

1. Remove the slide cartridges from storage.

2. Warm the wrapped cartridge at room temperature for 30 minute when taken from the refrigerator or 60 minutes from the freezer.

3. Unwrap and load the cartridge into the slide supply.

Measuring (Reportable or Dynamic) Range(mg/dL)**:**

Serum	-	1.00-14.00
Urine	-	1.00-17.80

STATISTICAL METHODS APPLIED:

Following statistical methods are applied in the present study.

1. **Crosstabs Procedures** (contingency coefficient test)

2. **Descriptive Statistics**

3. **Independent Samples 't' test**

A brief description of each statistical method is given below:

1. Crosstabs Procedures

The crosstabs procedures form two-way and multiway tables and provide a variety of tests and measures of association for two way tables. The structure of the table and the categories ordered determine what test or measure to use.

2. Descriptive Statistics

The descriptive procedure displays a univariate summary statistics for several variables in a single table and calculates standardized values (2-scores). Variables can be ordered by the size of their means (in ascending or descending order), alphabetically, or the order in which the variables are selected.

3. Independent Samples 't' test

The independent samples 't' test procedures compare the mean for two groups of cases. Ideally, for this test, the subject should be randomly assigned to two groups, so that any difference in response is due to treatment (or lack of treatment) and not to other factors. The statistics are done by using **SPSS** for windows packages version-16.

REVIEW OF LITERATURE

Pregnancy induced hypertension (PIH) are used to describe a condition in a wide spectrum of patients may have only minimal elevation in blood pressure or severe hypertension is the hallmark for the diagnosis of Preeclampsia. The elevation of blood pressure may be evident during the second trimester, early third trimester or at term. The manifestations in these patients are clinically similar but they result from several different underlying causes[37].

HISTORICAL ASPECTS:

Preeclampsia was reported back to nearly 2000 years when Celus reported an account of seizures in pregnant women that abated after delivery. This abnormality was given the name "Eclampsia", which in Greek means lightening, to describe its rapid and unexpected appearance[38].

Sometime during the middle of 1800s, examination of Urine for proteins in women with Eclampsia revealed severe proteinuria that antedated the seizures. In the latter part of the 1800s, when it became possible to measure blood pressure with a Sphygmomanometer, it further became apparent that eclamptic women also had high blood pressure, and like proteinuria this also antedated the seizures. As proteinuria and hypertension antedated Eclampsia, the term "Preeclampsia" was applied to the development of Hypertension and Proteinuria during gestation[39].

CLASSIFICATION OF HYPERTENSIVE DISORDERS OF PREGNANCY:

According to the American College of Obstetricians and Gynecologists (1996a), terminology used to describe hypertension in pregnancy is non uniform, confusing and steeped in tradition. Previously, the College had used the criteria of Hughes[40], and these are similar to those of Davey and McGillivray[41].

The working group of the National high blood pressure education program (NHBPEP) (1990) recommended that the original classification of **Hughes**[40] be used because "transient hypertension" is included. This corresponds to pregnancy induced hypertension without pathological edema or proteinuria[42].

Unfortunately no classification is adequate if etiology is unknown. Therefore frequently used classification is the modified classification of **American College of Obstetricians and Gynecologists** (1986), which is used here also[43].

The classification is as follows:

Classification of hypertensive disorders complicating pregnancy[43]:

1.   Pregnancy induced hypertension:

Hypertension that develops as a consequence of pregnancy and regresses postpartum which includes:

(A)   Hypertension without proteinuria or pathological edema

(B)   Preeclampsia is defined as hypertension with proteinuria and/or pathological edema occuring after 20 weeks; but going away by 12 weeks postpartum[44].

    I.   Mild   and   **II.**   Severe

(C)   Eclampsia with proteinuria and/or pathological edema along with convulsion

2.   <u>Coincidental hypertension</u>:

Chronic underlying hypertension that antedates pregnancy or persist postpartum

3.   <u>Pregnancy aggravated hypertension</u>:

Underlying hypertension worsened by pregnancy, this includes:

(a) Superimposed Preeclampsia

(b) Superimposed Eclampsia

4.   <u>Transient hypertension</u>:

Hypertension which develops after the mid trimester of pregnancy is characterized by mild elevations of Blood pressure that do not compromise the pregnancy. This form of hypertension regresses after delivery but may return in subsequent gestations. Predisposing factors are:

- Nulliparity
- Black race
- Maternal age below 20 or over 35 years

- Low socioeconomic status

- Multiple gestations

- Hydatidiform mole

- Polyhydramnios

- Non-immune fetal hydrops

- Twins

- Obesity

- Diabetes

- Chronic hypertension

- Underlying renal disease

Preeclampsia has been described as a disease of theories, because the cause is unknown. Some theories include:

(1)   Endothelial cell injury

(2)   Rejection phenomenon (insufficient production of blocking antibodies)

(3)   Compromised placental perfusion

(4)   Altered vascular reactivity

(5)   Imbalance between prostacyclin and thromboxane

(6)   Decreased glomerular filtration rate with retention of salt and water

(7)   Decreased intravascular volume

(8)   Increased central nervous system irritability

(9)   Disseminated intravascular coagulation

(10)   Uterine muscle stretch (ischemia)

(11)   Dietary factors

(12)   Genetic factors

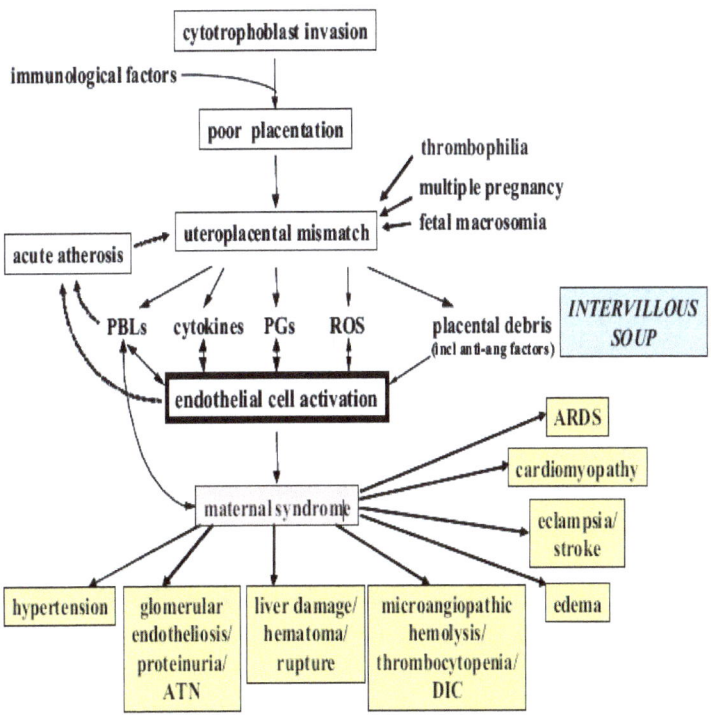

Figure 3: Pathophysiology of Preeclamsia

Anti-ANG Factors: Anti-Angiogenic Factors (e.g., s-Flt-1: PlGF ratio); **ARDS**: acute respiratory distress syndrome; **ATN**: Acute Tubular Necrosis; **DIC**: disseminated intravascular coagulation; **PBLs:** Peripheral Blood Leukocytes; **PGs**: Eicosanoids (e.g., TXA1:PGI2 ratio); **ROS**: Reactive Oxygen Species

The most popular theory for the pathogenesis of Preeclampsia describes a two-stage process, which ultimately results in a mismatch between uteroplacental supply and fetal demands, leading to maternal endothelial cell dysfunction and the maternal (and fetal) manifestations of Preeclampsia (Figure-1) [45 and 46].

Proteinuria is an important sign of toxemia. **Chesley**[47]rightfully concluded that diagnosis is questionable in its absence. Proteinuria is an important indicator of severity, because it usually develops late in the course of disease. Certainly persistent proteinuria of 2+ or more is severe Preeclampsia.

Vasospasm is basic to pathophysiology of Preeclampsia. Vascular constriction causes resistance to blood flow and accounts for the development of arterial hypertension.

Zeek and Assali[48]described obstructive changes in decidual vessels of patients with Preeclampsia, due to acute atherosis of spiral arterioles and venous lakes, no consistent lipid deposition has been substantiated and the Serum lipid levels have not be related to such events.

In summary, the current hypothesis for the pathogenesis of Preeclampsia is that an immunologic disturbance causes abnormal placental implantation resulting in decreased placental perfusion. The abnormal perfusion stimulates the production of substances in the blood that activate or injure endothelial cells. The vascular endothelium provides a single target for these blood-borne products, which explains the multiple organ system involvement in Preeclampsia.

Clinical Sequelae of Toxemia (and Preeclampsia):

The Kidney:

With hypertension in pregnancy, renal hemodynamic decrease by approximately 25% compared with normal pregnancy. Since renal hemodynamic increase 30 to 50% in normal gestation, the glomerular filtration rate and effective renal plasma flow toxemic women often remain above pre-pregnancy values.

The Liver:

Preeclampsia may also affect the liver, but this involvement is usually mild[49]. An exception is the variant, marked by signs of severe liver dysfunction combined with marked coagulation changes.

The Placenta:

Nourishing the foetus is a primary function of the placenta. When establishing hemochorial placentation, the non-villous trophoblast breaches the spiral arteries in the basal deciduas and later migrates down the arteries, reaching the radial arteries in the myometrium[50]. The interaction between endovascular trophoblasts and the tissues of the maternal vessel walls adapts these arteries to the vessels empty into the intervillous space. Loss of musculoelastic tissue results in dilated vessels; which permits increased blood flow into the intervillous space.

In toxaemia of pregnancy, placental blood flow, as determined by placental clearances, is reduced, with concomitant decrement in intervillous blood oxygen saturation. Obviously, there are several structural features that could cause or may be associated with reduced placental blood flow.

The Central Nervous System:

Eclampsia is the convulsive phase of Preeclampsia and may occur at any time prior to, during, or after delivery; as one third of the reported cases present on the first postpartum day. Hypertension and convulsions have been termed later postpartum Eclampsia, but whether or not these patients in fact had Preeclampsia is controversial[51].

Cerebral hemorrhage is the major cause of maternal death from toxemia (Preeclampsia or Eclampsia). As well as large hemorrhages, diffusely scattered infarcts, cortical petechiae, smaller subcortical hemorrhages, and necrotic arterioles (some containing fibrin thrombi) are found. The large hemorrhages are like those found in hypertension in nonpregnant individuals and the other changes are like the autopsy findings seen in hypertensive encephalopathy however, is not strictly correct because although Eclampsia usually correlates with the severity of the hypertension, it may also arise when blood pressure elevation are mild[49].

However, it is not unusual to observe a gravida who suddenly develops proteinuria and ever convulse over a short period of time even through the blood pressure differs little from that recorded 24 hours previously.

Table 7: Preeclampsia is further classified into mild and severe forms as follows[52]:

ABNORMALITY	MILD	SEVERE
Diastolic blood pressure	< 100 mm of Hg	≥ 110 mm of Hg
Proteinuria	Trace to +1, +2	Persistent ≥
Headache	Absent	Present
Visual disturbances	Absent	Present
Upper abdominal pain	Absent	Present
Oliguria	Absent	Present
Convulsions	Absent	Present in Eclampsia
Serum creatinine	Normal	Elevated
Thrombocytopenia	Absent	Present
Liver enzyme Elevation	Minimal	Marked
Fetal growth restriction	Absent	Obvious
Pulmonary edema	Absent	Present

ETIOLOGY AND PATHOGENESIS OF PREECLAMPSIA[52]:

1. Immunological factors :

There is circumstantial evidence to support the theory that Preeclampsia is immune mediated. **Dekker GA and Sibi BM** (1998) in their article "Etiology and pathogenesis of Preeclampsia: current concepts" reviewed that in the early second trimester, women destined to develop Preeclampsia have a significantly lower proportion of helper T cells (Th1) compared with that of women who remain normotensive[53].

Hayashi M et al (2005) in their article "Elevation of granulocyte colony stimulating factor in the placenta and blood in Preeclampsia" stated that these helper T lymphocytes secrete specific cytokines that promote implantation and their dysfunction mayfavorPreeclampsia[54].

2. Inflammatory factors :

Gervasi MT et al (2001) in their article "Phenotype and metabolic characteristics of monocytes and granulocytes in Preeclampsia" reviewed that Preeclampsia is considered a disease due to an extreme state of activated leukocytes in the maternal circulation. Cytokines such as tumor necrosis factor-α (TNF-α) and the interleukins may contribute to the oxidative stress associated with Preeclampsia[55].

3. Genetic factors :

Chesley LC and Copper DW (1986) in the article "Genetics of hypertension in pregnancy; Possible single gene control of Preeclampsia and Eclampsia in the descendents of eclamptic women" concluded that single gene hypothesis fits well but multifactorial inheritance cannot be excluded[56].

Ners PB et al (2003) in the article "Family history of hypertension, heart disease and stroke among woman who developed hypertension" predicted that the hereditary hypertension undoubtedly is linked to Preeclampsia, and the tendency for Preeclampsia–Eclampsia is inherited[57].

4. Dietary factors :

John JH et al (2002) in the article 'Effects of fruit and vegetable consumption on plasma antioxidant concentrations and blood pressure: A randomized controlled trail" showed that in the general population a diet high in fruits and vegetables that have antioxidant activity is associated with decreased blood pressure[58].

Marcoux S et al (1991) in the article "Calcium intake from dairy products and supplements and the risks of Preeclampsia and gestational hypertension" reported that after mid pregnancy dietary supplementation with 2g of elemental Calcium per day significantly reduced the incidence of hypertension[59].

CALCIUM:

Calcium is the fifth most common element, and the most prevalent cation, in the body. An average human body contains approximately 1 kg (24.95mol) of Calcium. Calcium is found in three main compartments, the skeleton, soft tissue and extracellular fluid. The skeleton contains 99% of the body's Calcium, predominantly as extracellular crystals of unknown structure with a composition approaching that of hydroxyapatite[60].

In blood, virtually all of the Calcium is in the plasma, which has a mean normal Calcium concentration of approximately 9.5 mg/dL (2.38 mmol/L) Calcium exists in three physiochemical states in plasma of which approximately 50% is free (ionized), 40% is bound to plasma proteins and 10% is complexed with small ions[60].

The free Calcium fraction is the biologically active form; its concentration in plasma is tightly regulated by the Calcium regulating hormones, Parathyroid hormone and 1, 25 dihydroxycholecalciferol. About 80% of protein bound Calcium is associated with albumin with the remaining 20% associated with globulins[60].

Extracellular Calcium provides Calcium ion for the maintenance of intracellular Calcium, bone mineralization, blood coagulation and plasma membrane potential. Calcium stabilizes the plasma membranes and influences permeability and excitability[43].

A decrease in the free Serum Calcium concentration causes increased neuromuscular excitability and tetany. An increased Serum Calcium concentration reduces neuromuscular excitability[60].

Physiologic Changes in Calcium Metabolism during Pregnancy:

Calcium is an essential nutrient during pregnancy and lactation. Calcium contributes to bone development in the fetus and neonate and is considered a critical nutrient. Physiological changes in Calcium metabolism occur during pregnancy and lactation. Some women may lose some of their bone density during pregnancy and/or lactation. For all women, pregnancy and lactation are times of high Calcium requirement. The average Calcium demand of a developing fetus is 30 g by the end of gestation[61]. Eighty percent of this Calcium amount is acquired during the third trimester while the fetal skeleton is rapidly developing[61]. The average Calcium transfer to the fetus during pregnancy is 50 mg/day during the second trimester and 250 mg/day during the third trimester[62].

One of the earliest changes in Calcium metabolism during pregnancy is a decrease in total Serum Calcium. This change is not physiologically significant though, and can be attributed to the decrease in Serum albumin and the normal hemodilution that occurs during pregnancy. Levels of ionized Calcium stay in the normal range. PTH levels fall into a low-normal range during the first trimester, but rise throughout the pregnancy to reach normal levels by the end of gestation. Calcitonin levels are increased throughout pregnancy, preventing extreme Calcium loss from the maternal skeleton.

Urinary Calcium excretion tends to increase across the course of pregnancy, from 12 weeks gestation onward, and can be associated with the increase in intestinal absorption, increased related filtered load of Calcium, and the increased glomerular filtration rate that occurs during pregnancy[61].

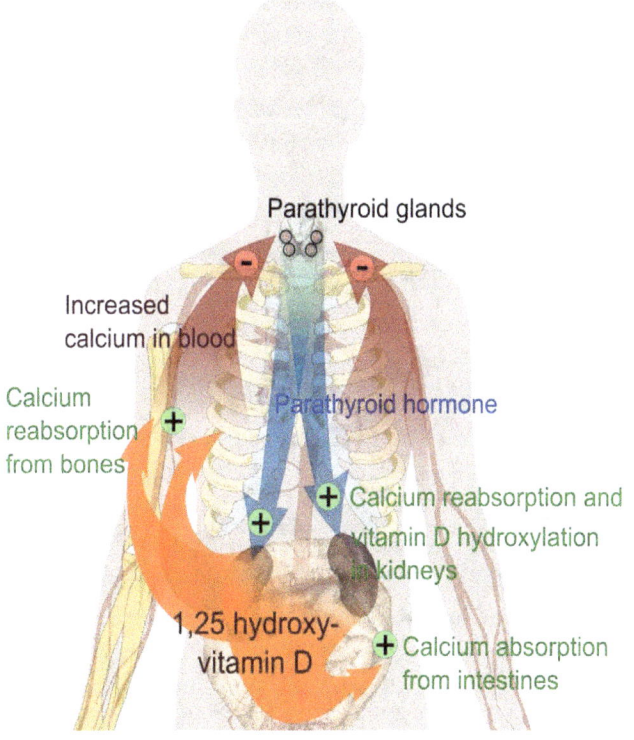

Figure 4: Calcium metabolism

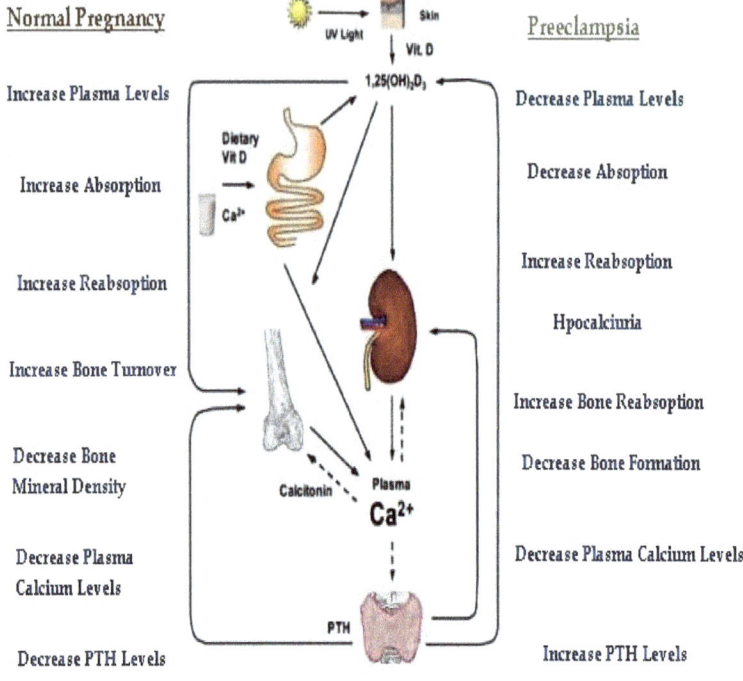

Normal Pregnancy

Increase Plasma Levels

Increase Absorption

Increase Reabsoption

Increase Bone Turnover

Decrease Bone
Mineral Density

Decrease Plasma
Calcium Levels

Decrease PTH Levels

Preeclampsia

Decrease Plasma Levels

Decrease Absoption

Increase Reabsoption

Hpocalciuria

Increase Bone Reabsoption

Decrease Bone Formation

Decrease Plasma Calcium Levels

Increase PTH Levels

Figure 5: Calcium metabolism in Pregnancy and Preeclampsia

In summary, the extra demand for Calcium from the growing fetus, especially during the third trimester, is physiologically compensated through changes in hormone levels. These hormonal changes lead to an increase in intestinal absorption, a decrease in renal Calcium loss, and an increase in absorption from the maternal skeleton (intestinal Calcium absorption becoming the primary source).

Calcium Intake and Hypertensive Disorders:

Several studies have examined whether Calcium supplements would help reduce the incidence of pregnancy induced hypertension and Preeclampsia. This idea first developed because of a 1980 epidemiological study conducted in Guatemala where scientists noticed that the Mayan Indians exhibited high Calcium intakes and low incidences of Preeclampsia and Eclampsia[63].

Eclampsia is more common in countries where the dietary Calcium intake is low. Additionally, observational studies in the U.S. and Canada have shown that women who have lower Calcium intakes exhibit a greater incidence of pregnancy induced hypertension[64].

The physiological basis behind this hypothesis is that low Calcium intake stimulates PTH production, which increases the intracellular Calcium levels. This leads to smooth-muscle vessel contraction and hypertension. Calcium supplements would reduce the intracellular Calcium and relax the vessels[63].

Atallah et al (2004)[63] conducted a review of research on the effects of Calcium supplementation in PIH and Preeclampsia. They found that, among 11 studies, 10 demonstrated a reduction in the incidence of hypertension with additional dietary Calcium. Calcium supplements seemed to reduce the risk of PIH and Preeclampsia in women who were at high risk for developing gestational hypertension. This reduction occurred among teenagers; women over 35 years old; African Americans; women with multiple gestation, preexisting diabetes, hypertension, renal disease, or obesity; and women with a personal or family history of PIH or Preeclampsia[65]. Calcium supplementation also reduced the incidence of PIH and Preeclampsia in women with low dietary Calcium intake[63].

One study that did not find a difference in hypertension with the use of Calcium was a large research study conducted in the U.S. with 4,589 healthy, pregnant women. In this particular study, women were given either 2 g/day of supplemental Calcium or a placebo, starting anywhere from 13 to 21 weeks gestation. The researchers Levine R J et al[66] (1997) found the systolic and diastolic blood pressures were similar in each group, and the increase in Calcium did not reduce any of the consequences of Preeclampsia and PIH (e.g., preterm deliveries, small-for-gestational-age infants, or infant fatalities). Additionally, the frequency of Eclampsia and HELLP syndrome (Hemolysis, Elevated Liver enzymes, and Low Platelet count) was almost equal in both groups.

However, the results from many clinical studies show the relationship between the aggravation of hypertensive complication and changes in concentration of various chemicals in mother's Serum. Interestingly, the significant reduction in Serum Calcium and Magnesium are found in preeclamptic mothers[6].

Possible metabolic abnormalities include a decrease in Serum 1, 25-dihydroxycholecalciferol concentration, a decrease in Serum ionized Calcium concentration and a decrease in urinary Calcium excretion[67and68].

An increase in intracellular Calcium in vascular smooth muscle cells during pregnancy is consistent with development of vasoconstriction and resultant hypertension[69].

The biochemical mechanism responsible for the possible increase in intracellular Calcium and concomitant decrease in extracellular Calcium is presently unclear. Also, it has been suggested that parathyroid hormone plays a crucial role in influencing Calcium transport. Unfortunately studies of parathyroid hormone concentration during uncomplicated and hypertensive pregnancies have been inconclusive[70].

The recommended dietary allowance (RDA) for Calcium varies with age and, for adults, with gender. Recommended dietary allowance value for adults starts at 1000 mg per day. Urine Calcium levels will reflect dietary intake. In average adult Urine sample collected over 24 hours, 100-250 mg of Calcium (2.50-6.25 mmol) is expected. For those on low-Calcium diets 50-150 mg/day is expected, while those on a Calcium-free diet will have 5-40 mg/day. It is also important to note that Calcium excretion is heavily influenced by sodium excretion. Low-sodium diets tend to decrease Calcium excretion and vice versa[71].

Measurement of total Calcium[60]:

Many methods have been used historically to measure total Calcium. Today, only photometric, Ion Selective Electrode and occasionally atomic absorption spectrophotometry methods are routinely used by clinical laboratories for the measurement of Serum and Urine total Calcium. According to the College of American pathologist comprehensive chemistry survey, in 2004 approximately 79% of participating clinical laboratories used photometric methods 35% Arsenezo III, 44% Cresolphthalein Complexone and 20% of laboratories used Ion Selective Electrode methods for total Serum

Calcium. Ion Selective Electrode for the measurements of total Calcium was introduced more recently than photometric methods. Analyzers using Ion Selective Electrodes capable of providing immediate whole blood determination of free Calcium are now widely available.

The reference intervals for total and free Calcium in Serum and plasma of adults:

Total Calcium : 8.6 to 10.2 mg/dL (2.15 to 2.55 mmol/L)

Free Calcium (ionized) : 4.6 to 5.3 mg/dL (1.15 to 1.33 mmol/L)

MAGNESIUM:

Magnesium is the fourth most abundant cation in the body and the second most prevalent intracellular cation. In humans, less than 1% of total body Magnesium is found in Serum and red blood cells. It is distributed principally between bone (53%) muscle (27%) and soft tissue (19%). Serum Magnesium comprises only about 0.3% of total Magnesium, where it is present in 3 states – ionized (62%), protein bound (30%) mainly to albumin and complexed to anions such as citrate and phosphate. Rich sources of Magnesium in the diet include cereals and legumes. Magnesium absorption occurs principally from the ileum and colon. Excretion of Magnesium occurs via the kidney[72].

Magnesium is the cofactor for more than 300 enzymes in the body. It is required for enzyme substrate formation (for example Magnesium ATP). In addition, Magnesium is an allosteric activator of many enzyme systems. Examples of enzymes that require Magnesium for action include adenylate cyclase, Na+-K+ adenosine triphosphate (ATPase), Ca2+-ATPase, phosphofructokinase and creatine kinase.

Magnesium is important in oxidative phosphorylation, glycolysis, cell replication, nucleotide metabolism and protein biosynthesis[60].

Pregnancy is a state of Magnesium depletion. The total and ionized Magnesium levels are significantly lower in normal pregnancy compared to non-pregnant women. The levels tend to fall during pregnancy and further decrease in women who develop Preeclampsia later. It is also mentioned in previous studies that the concentration of Magnesium during pregnancy exceeds the intake creating a state of physiological hypomagnesaemia.

Although, the definitive treatment of Preeclampsia includes delivery of the fetus and placenta, Magnesium sulphate is the modality of choice for prevention and treatment of eclamptic seizures. Currently there is better understanding of the mechanisms of action of Magnesium sulphate in regulating the neuromuscular excitability by acting directly on the myoneural junction and antagonizing N-methyl-D-aspartate receptor activation. The presynaptic release of acetylcholine is also reduced, thereby altering neuromuscular transmission. Dilatation of cerebral blood vessels takes place thus reducing cerebral ischemia. Also the peripheral arteriolar dilatation reduces the blood pressure. The precise mechanism of action for the tocolytic effects may be related to the action of Magnesium as a Calcium blocker thus inhibiting muscle contractions[73].

Generally, the hypomagnesaemia in most pregnant women is associated with hemodilution, renal clearance during pregnancy and consumption of minerals by the growing fetus. Recent studies report a relationship between hypomagnesaemia and pregnancy induced hypertension. Although the explanation for this result is not clear, they propose that Magnesium promotes vascular muscle relaxation. But, this result is contradictory to some studies which report that the mean Serum Magnesium level in Preeclampsia is not different from that of normal pregnancy[6].

Magnesium has been shown to improve endothelial function in Preeclampsia. This may be due to the direct vasodilating properties of Magnesium to stimulate, the release of endothelial vasodilators like prostacyclin which induces vasodilatation as well as inhibits platelet adherence and aggregation[74 and 75].

Preeclampsia has been treated with Magnesium salts since the turn of the century. Acute Magnesium sulphate administration elicits a rapid fall in systemic vascular resistance, and rise in cardiac index and a transient fall in blood pressure[76 and 77].

Magnesium sulphate infusion also increases renal blood flow and stimulates production and release of prostacyclin in Preeclampsia but not in preterm labour[75 and 78].

The reference interval for total Serum Magnesium in adult is 1.7 to 2.4mg/dL (0.66to 1.08mmol/L). Magnesium concentration in erythrocytes is approximately three times that of Serum.

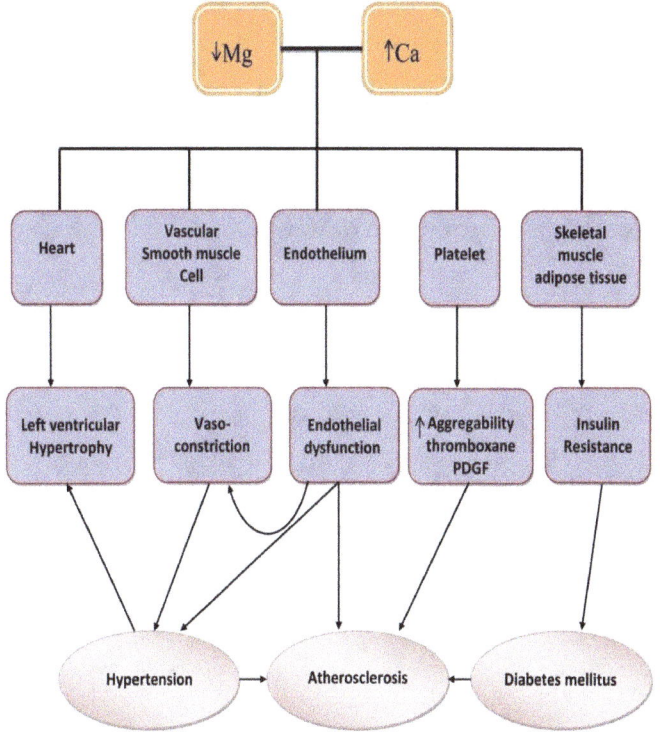

Figure 6: Role of Magnesium and Calcium in the pathophysiology of Hypertension, Diabetes mellitus and Atherosclerosis.

URIC ACID:

In humans, Uric acid (2,6,8-trihydroxypurine) is the major product of the catabolism of the purine nucleosides adenosine and guanosine. Purines formed from the catabolism of dietary nucleic acids are converted to Uric acid directly. The bulk of purine excreted as Uric acid arises from degradation of endogenous nucleic acid. The rate of synthesis of Uric acid is approximately 400 mg per day; dietary sources contribute another 300mg[79].

Uric acid is a product of purine degradation catalyzed by the enzyme xanthine dehydrogenase/xanthine oxidase (XDH/XO). XDH is converted to its oxidase form XO by several stimuli including ischemia[80]. Purine metabolism by XO couples the production of Uric acid with the production of the free radical superoxide (O_2^-), and is implicated as a contributor to oxidative stress[80]. XDH/XO is found in most tissues but is concentrated in the liver and gut. Recently, a circulating population of XO has been identified that increases dramatically following ischemic tissue damage[81]. Increased circulating Uric acid accompanies similar insults[82]. It is speculated that circulating XO can bind to endothelium and lead to local oxidative injury[83].

Uric acid is minimally soluble and its concentration is maintained relatively low in healthy individuals (<6.0 mg/dL). However, even low concentrations of Uric acid possess biological function. Uric acid is a plasma antioxidant capable of scavenging superoxide, hydroxyl radical and singlet oxygen[84].

Uric Acid during Pregnancy:

Uric acid concentrations are influenced by diet (i.e. high protein, and fructose), alcohol consumption, and increased cell turnover, enzymatic defects in purine metabolism or altered kidney function[85]. Estrogen is uricosuric and Uric acid concentrations are higher in men and post-menopausal women[86]. In pregnancy Uric acid concentrations initially fall 25-35% due to the effects of estrogen, expanded blood volume and increased glomerular filtration rate[87]. However, concentrations slowly rise to those observed in non-pregnant women by term gestation (4-6 mg/dL)[88].

Hyperuricemia and Preeclampsia:

Elevated Uric acid concentrations were first noted in preeclamptic women in the late 1800s. Since that time numerous reports have demonstrated a relationship between Uric acid concentrations and severity of disease[89and90]. Nonetheless, the clinical utility of hyperuricemia in the management of Preeclampsia is controversial. Recently we examined the relationship of high Uric acid elevations in pregnant hypertensive women to the endpoints of preterm birth (largely indicated preterm birth for the management of Preeclampsia) and growth restriction[90]. Hyperuricemia was present in 16% of women with gestational hypertension without proteinuria and 75% of women with clinically diagnosed PE. Pregnancy hypertension with hyperuricemia was associated with an excess of these adverse fetal outcomes. The increased frequency of preterm birth and growth restriction was present in hypertensive women with elevated concentration of Uric acid even in the absence of proteinuria.

In women who go on to develop Preeclampsia, Uric acid concentration is elevated as early as 10 weeks of gestation, a time much earlier than the clinical presentation of the disorder. Increased Uric acid often precedes clinical manifestations of the disease, including reduced glomerular filtration rate[90]. Nonetheless, hyperuricemia has historically been attributed to reduced renal clearance. Uric acid is filtered, reabsorbed and secreted by the kidney. Hypovolumia, an early change in Preeclampsia, increases Uric acid reabsorption which could increase Serum Uric acid concentrations. However, increased Uric acid precedes the reduction in plasma volume[91]. Increased Uric acid production from maternal, fetal or placental tissues through heightened tissues breakdown (i.e. increased substrate availability) and/or increased XO activity could also explain the increased concentration. The possible roles of placental ischemia-reperfusion injury, reduced antioxidant capacity and oxidative stress will be discussed below.

Uric Acid as a Pathogenic Vascular Factor:

Evidence for a pathogenic role of Uric acid is increasing. In the non-pregnant population hyperuricemia is an independent predictor of cardiovascular and renal disease in both the general population and in subjects with chronic hypertension. Uric acid is also a marker for adverse cardiovascular events in patients with established cardiovascular disease[85].

Summary:

Hyperuricemia is one of the earliest and most consistent observations noted in preeclamptic pregnancies. While elevated concentrations of circulating Uric acid are not uniformly seen in every woman with Preeclampsia, they do appear to identify a subset of preeclamptic women who are at greater risk for maternal and fetal morbidities. Also, hyperuricemia in pregnant women without proteinuria is at least as good a predictor of fetal morbidity as hypertension and proteinuria.

We speculate that Uric acid may play direct roles in the pathological processes of Preeclampsia at both the level of the placenta and maternal vasculature. The evidence used to formulate this hypothesis was drawn heavily from epidemiological and clinical studies of non-pregnant individuals describing positive associations between hyperuricemia and risk of cardiovascular events, in addition to work demonstrating an independent association between elevated Uric acid and poor fetal outcome. The hypothesis is further supported by in-vitro culture studies and hyperuricemia animal models demonstrating several pathogenic effects of Uric acid, including pro-inflammatory effects, stimulation of smooth muscle cell proliferation, inhibition of endothelial cell proliferation and migration, promotion of endothelial dysfunction and damage. These insults all play pivotal roles in the pathophysiology of Preeclampsia. We propose that there is sufficient evidence to support a pathogenic role for Uric acid in this disorder that warrants further investigation[92].

CALCIUM/CREATININE RATIO:

It was observed that there is hypocalciuria in pregnancy induced hypertension and suggested that these changes could be partly related to decrease in GFR in Preeclampsia but tubular reabsorption was also reduced because the fractional excretion of Calcium was decreased[93].

Urine Creatinine is a known marker of renal function. Excretion of Calcium & Creatinine is affected by the factors which influence functions of the kidneys. Normal Urinary Calcium concentration is 100 to 300 mg/24 hours. Normal Urinary Creatinine concentration is 1500 to 3000 mg/24 hours. Although a 24-hour collection is best, random Urine Calcium measurement can be performed and is expressed in relation to Creatinine. A normal reference interval for the Urinary Calcium/Creatinine ratio is <0.14[71].

Taufield P et al (1987) in the study "Hypocalciuria in Preeclampsia" observed that urinary Calcium excretion averaged 313±140 mg/day in a normal pregnant woman, 248±139 mg/day in those with transient hypertension and 223±41 mg/day in those with chronic hypertension. Calcium excretion in women with Preeclampsia was 42 ± 29 mg/day and in chronic hypertension with superimposed Preeclampsia it was 78±49 mg/day. It was concluded that measurement of urinary Calcium might be useful in distinguishing Preeclampsia from other forms of gestational hypertension[94].

Huikeshoven FJM et al (1990) in the study "Hypocalciuria in Hypertensive Disorder of Pregnancy and How to Measure It" in 41 women in the third trimester; found that there is a significant decrease in 24 hour Calcium excretion in hypertensive and preeclamptic subjects. It was found mild hypocalciuria in women with gestational hypertension without proteinuria. The hypocalciuria in women with Preeclampsia was associated with a decreased fractional excretion of Calcium and concluded that measurement of Calcium excretion may be useful in predicting Pregnancy induced hypertension[95].

Vural P et al (2000) in the study "Calcium and Phosphate Excretion in Preeclampsia" stated that Hypocalciuria and hypophosphateuria were found to be important features of severe Preeclampsia and probably indirectly are related to the altered renal function seen in toxemia of pregnancy[96].

Ramos et al (1991) have found that the patients with Preeclampsia had reduced urinary excretion of Calcium; suggesting that Calcium measurement may be useful in screening for this condition[26 and 28].

Sheela CN et al (2011) in the study "Calcium/Creatinine Ratio and Microalbuminuria in Prediction of Preeclampsia" said that Calcium/Creatinine Ratio at 0.04 in spot Urine sample being a good test for prediction of Preeclampsia can be recommended as a screening test in all asymptomatic pregnant women, for Preeclampsia {p-value<0.001 (strongly significant)}. Microalbuminuria does not seem to be effective as a screening tool for Preeclampsia at present[36].

Kazerooni T et al (2003) in the study "Calcium/Creatinine Ratio in a Spot sample of Urine for Early Prediction of Preeclampsia" found that single Urine Calcium to creatinine ratio {p-value<0.03 (moderately significant)} may be an effective method for screening women at greatest risk for Preeclampsia[97].

Rodriguez MH et al (1988) in the article "Calcium/Creatinine Ratio and Microalbuminuria in the Prediction of Preeclampsia" stated that changes in renal function are present in gravid women who are otherwise free of symptoms in which Preeclampsia will eventually develop. Testing for microalbuminuria and a Calcium/Creatinine Ratio may be a useful screening tool in predicting the subsequent development of Preeclampsia[20].

Saudan PJ et al (1998) in the article "Urinary Calcium/Creatinine Ratio as a Predictor of Preeclampsia" stated that Calcium/Creatinine Ratio measurement does not have sufficient sensitivity to recommend its use as a screening test for the emergence of Preeclampsia[98].

Ozcan T et al (1995) in the study "Urinary Calcium/Creatinine Ratio for Predicting Preeclampsia" found that a single Urine Calcium to creatinine ratio {p-value<0.0001 (strongly significant)} might be an effective marker for predicting Preeclampsia in a high risk population[99].

Phuapradit W et al (1993) in the study "Urinary Calcium/Creatinine Ratio in the Prediction of Preeclampsia" found that the patients with Preeclampsia did not have significantly less excretion of Calcium than the normotensives[100].

Kazemi AFN et al (2010) in the article " The Predictive Value of Urinary Calcium to Creatinine Ratio, Roll-Over Test and BMI in Early Diagnosis of Preeclampsia" stated that Calcium to creatinine ratio, BMI and ROT test did not accurate if done as a separate test for prediction of Preeclampsia but the clinical usability of those test are significant in Preeclampsia control; so it is advised to use these cheap and low risk tests specially in 28-32 weeks of pregnancy for screening Preeclampsia[101].

Ye Y et al (1995) in the article "Predictive Value of Urinary Calcium Measurement on Occurrence of Pregnancy Induced Hypertension" stated that Low urinary Calcium excretion is a valuable marker for prediction of PIH[102].

Suzuki Y et al (1992) in the article "Urinary Calcium Excretion as an Early Prediction Marker for Pregnancy Induced Hypertension" stated that urinary Calcium/Creatinine Ratio was significantly lower in the women with PIH than in the healthy pregnant women, and it was especially low in those with Pregnancy Induced Hypertension who had no family history of hypertension[103].

Kar J et al (2002) have shown that a single Urinary Calcium/Creatinine Ratio may be an effective screening method for impending Preeclampsia and may identify population at greater risk to be included in primary prevention programmes[104].

Baker PN et al (1994) have shown that low Urinary Calcium/Creatinine Ratio may be a useful screening tool between 24 to 34 weeks of gestation for predicting the development of Preeclampsia in asymptomatic patients[105].

Moni SY et al (2009) in the article "Role of Calcium Therapy on Urinary Calcium/Creatinine Ratio in Healthy Pregnant Women and preeclamptic Women" stated that Urinary Calcium/Creatinine Ratio was within normal range in healthy pregnant women and after Calcium therapy this ratio was not significantly changed. On the other hand urinary Calcium/Creatinine Ratio in PET women was significantly decreased and this ratio was significantly increased after Calcium therapy. These observations suggest that low Urinary Calcium/Creatinine Ratio help in early prediction of PET and Calcium supplement during pregnancy may reduce the incidence of PET[106].

McGrowder D et al (2009) in the study "Hypocalciuria in Preeclampsia and Gestational Hypertension due to Decreased Fractional Excretion of Calcium" found that a lower urinary Calcium-to-creatinine ratio (0.17±0.03) in preeclamptic women compared with normotensive women (0.45±0.08)[107].

Raniolo E et al (1993) in the study "Prediction of PIH By Means of Urinary Calcium Creatinine Ratio" stated that the mean Urinary Calcium/Creatinine Ratio with normotensive pregnancies was 0.52 (SD 0.32) which was not significantly different from those who developed Preeclampsia 0.49 (SD 0.32) or gestational hypertension 0.57 (SD 0.41)[108].

Suarez VR et al (1996) in the article "Urinary Calcium is Asymptomatic Primigravidas who later developed Preeclampsia" found that 24 hour urinary Calcium excretion between 17 and 20 weeks in primigravidae was studied. Using a cut off level of 3.4 mg/kg/24 hours the sensitivity was 80%, specificity was 64.8%, positive predictive value was 38.7% and the negative predictive value was 92.1%[27].

Kamra R et al (1994) in the article "Role of Urinary Calcium/Creatinine Ratio in the Prediction of Pregnancy Induced Hypertension" found that the Calcium/Creatinine Ratio of <0.04 in 13.46% patients of whom 71.4% developed PIH, which was statistically highly significant, with an Odds ratio of 53.75, sensitivity – 71.4%, specificity – 95.5%, positive predictive value –71.4% and negative predictive value – 95.5%[109].

Sukonpan K et al (2005) in the study "Serum Calcium and Serum Magnesium in Normal and preeclamptic Pregnancy" found that both Serum Calcium and Serum Magnesium levels in preeclamptic pregnant women are lower than in normal pregnant women. These findings support the hypothesis that hypocalcaemia and hypomagnesaemia are possible etiologies of Preeclampsia[6].

Roodsari V et al (2008) in the article "Serum Calcium and Magnesium in preeclamptic and Normal Pregnancies: A Comparative Study" stated that Serum Magnesium level in Preeclampsia is lower than that of the normal pregnant women. This result may support the hypothesis on the role of Magnesium deficiency in Preeclampsia pathophysiology and suggest the usefulness of its assessment in the early diagnosis of the disorder[7].

Chanvitya P et al (2008) in the study "Serum Calcium, Magnesium and Uric acid in Preeclampsia and Normal Pregnancy" found that Serum Calcium in severe preeclamptic women was lower and Serum Uric acid was higher than normal pregnant women and mild preeclamptic women respectively but there was no difference between normal pregnant women and mild preeclamptic women. There was no difference in Serum Magnesium among normal pregnancy and both groups of Preeclampsia. These findings support that hypocalcaemia and hyperuricemia correlate to severe Preeclampsia[30].

K Kisters et al (1998) in the article "Plasma and Membrane Calcium and Magnesium Concentrations in Normal Pregnancy and in Preeclampsia" stated that lowered plasma and membrane Magnesium concentrations in Preeclampsia may contribute to the development of hypertension in pregnancy. Additionally, a disturbed Calcium homeostasis is observed in Preeclampsia[110].

Alavi A et al (2012) in the article "Comparison of Serum Calcium, Total Protein and Uric Acid Levels between Hypertensive and Healthy Pregnant Women in an Iranian Population" stated that Mean Serum Calcium level was significantly lower in hypertensive pregnant women in comparison with healthy ones. Considering this factor in prenatal care is important[111].

Kosch M et al (2000) in the article "Alterations of Plasma Calcium and Intracellular and Membrane Calcium in Erythrocytes of Patients with Preeclampsia" stated that membrane Calcium content is significantly increased in preeclamptic women despite low plasma Calcium concentrations. This finding suggests an altered membrane ion transport and may be of importance for the pathogenesis of Preeclampsia[112].

Malas NO et al (2001) in the article "Does Serum Calcium in Preeclampsia and Normal Pregnancy Differ?" stated that the low level of maternal total Calcium may have a role in the development of this disorder in pregnancy, therefore Calcium supplementation during late pregnancy may be used to help in the prevention of this disorder[113].

Cunha AR et al (2012) in the article "Magnesium and Vascular Changes in Hypertension" stated that Magnesium is a mineral with important functions in the body, and it is important that their levels are adequate. The conflicting results of studies evaluating the effects of Magnesium supplements on blood pressure and other cardiovascular outcomes indicate that the action of Magnesium in the vascular system is present but not yet established[114].

Sukonpan K et al (2005) in the article "Serum Calcium and Serum Magnesium in Normal and preeclamptic Pregnancies" stated that decrease in Serum Magnesium levels in preeclamptic patients when compared to the control group. Generally, the hypomagnesaemia in most pregnant women is associated with hemodilution, renal clearance during pregnancy and consumption of minerals by the growing fetus[6].

Touyz RM (2003) in the article "Role of Magnesium in the Pathogenesis of Hypertension" stated that the clinical aspect which has demonstrated the greatest therapeutic potential for Magnesium in hypertension is in the treatment of Preeclampsia and Eclampsia[115].

Seydoux J et al (1992) in the article "Serum and Intracellular Magnesium during Normal Pregnancy and in Patients with Preeclampsia" stated that there was a progressive reduction in total Serum Magnesium concentrations during normal pregnancy, thought to be partly due to hemodilution, because the decline in concentration of Serum proteins paralleled that of Magnesium (P less than 0.001). Their data does not support the conclusion that Magnesium deficiency is the primary cause of Preeclampsia[116].

Sayyed AK et al (2013) in the article "Electrolyte Status in Preeclampsia" stated that the study shows reduced levels of Serum Calcium, Magnesium, Potassium and increased level of sodium in patients of Preeclampsia as compared to the normal pregnant women. Hypocalcaemia, hypomagnesaemia, hypokalemia and hypernatremia seen in the preeclamptic women may be responsible for the vascular pathology associated with onset of Preeclampsia. Hence adjuvant supplementation of Calcium, Magnesium, and Potassium with dietary restriction of sodium may prevent further progression of Preeclampsia[117].

Chaurasia PP et al (2012) in the article "Changes in Serum Calcium and Serum Magnesium Level in preeclamptic Vs. Normal Pregnancy" stated that the Serum Calcium and Magnesium in preeclamptic women were $(8.9\pm0.4$ mg/dL vs. 9.7 ± 0.7 mg/dL, $p<0.0001)$ and $(0.75\pm0.08$ mmol/l vs. 0.85 ± 0.09 mmol/l, $p=0.001)$ respectively, significantly lower than that in normal pregnant women. These findings support the hypothesis that hypocalcaemia and hypomagnesaemia are possible etiologies of Preeclampsia[29].

Sendhav S et al (2013) in the article "A Comparative Study of Serum Uric Acid, Calcium and Magnesium in Preeclampsia and Normal Pregnancy" stated that they found significantly high Uric acid levels in severe preeclamptic women as compared with normal pregnant and mild preeclamptic women (p-value<0.05). Also there is significantly low Serum Magnesium and Serum Calcium levels in severe preeclamptic women as compared to normal pregnant and mild preeclamptic women (p-value<0.05). There was no significant difference found between normal and mild preeclamptic women[118].

Weerasekera DS (2003) in the article "The Significance of Serum Uric Acid, Creatinine and Urinary Microprotein Levels in Predicting Preeclampsia" stated that microproteinuria of more than 375 mg/L may be used as a cut-off value and as a screening test for the early detection of women at risk of developing Preeclampsia. Serum Uric acid and creatinine had no predictive value as a screening test for Preeclampsia[119].

Thangaratinam S et al (2006) in the study "Accuracy of Serum Uric Acid in Predicting Complications of Preeclampsia: A Systematic Review" found that Serum Uric acid is a poor predictor of maternal and fetal complications in women with Preeclampsia[120].

Kang et al (2004) in the article "Uric Acid, Endothelial Dysfunction and Preeclampsia" hypothesize that hyperuricemia may also have a contributory role in the development of hypertension and renal disease in these patients, and we review recent experimental data that would support this hypothesis[121].

Lam C et al (2005) in the article "Uric Acid and Preeclampsia" stated that this article reviews our current understanding of hyperuricemia in the setting of Preeclampsia, and highlights the hypothesis that hyperuricemia may contribute to vascular damage in Preeclampsia[122].

Sahijwani D et al (2012) in the article "Serum Uric Acid as a Prognostic Marker of Pregnancy Induced Hypertension" stated that Serum Uric acid >6mg/dL is associated with increased maternal complications specially Eclampsia and higher incidence of low birth weight[123].

OBSERVATIONS AND RESULTS

The present study analyses Urinary Calcium/Creatinine Ratio in 100 asymptomatic, normotensive pregnant women between 20-28 weeks gestation. Study also analyses the Serum levels of Calcium, Magnesium, and Uric acid in Preeclamptic women in third trimester in comparison with normal pregnant women taken as Controls.

ANALYSIS OF URINARY CALCIUM/CREATININE RATIO IN ASYMPTOMATIC, NORMOTENSIVE PREGNANT WOMEN BETWEEN 20-28 WEEKS GESTATION:

TABLE 8: Age wise distribution of Preeclamptic group and Control groups

Age (Years)	Preeclamptic Group	Control Group
20-24	07	44
25-29	05	41
30-35	01	02
Total	13	87
Mean age	24.77	24.91

The Mean age in the Preeclamptic group and Control group were 24.77 years and 24.91 years respectively. In the Preeclamptic group 53.84% and in the Control group 50.57% belonged to the age between 20-24 years. In the Preeclamptic group 38.46% and in the Control group 47.12% belonged to the age between 25-29 years. In the Preeclamptic group 14.28% and in the Control group 2.29% belonged to age group of 30-35 years.

TABLE 9: Clinical and Laboratory Characteristics of Study Groups

S.N.	Characteristics (Mean±SD)	Pre-eclamptic Women (N = 13)	Normo-tensive Women (N = 87)
1.	Mean Maternal Age (in years)	24.77±3.19	24.91±2.56
2.	Mean Gestational Age (in weeks) [at the time of joining the study]	25.08±2.40	25.15±2.63
3.	Systolic B.P. (mm of Hg) [at the time of joining the study]	119.69±7.52	117.43±7.58
4.	Diastolic B.P. (mm of Hg) [at the time of joining the study]	78.31±3.73	77.24±4.74
5.	Systolic B.P. (mm of Hg) [at the time delivery]	144.46±4.91	122.46±7.09
6.	Diastolic B.P. (mm of Hg) [at the time of delivery]	96.00±4.47	78.46±3.97
7.	Mean Urinary Calcium level (mg/dL)	4.56±1.19	9.23±3.49
8.	Mean Urinary Creatinine level (mg/dL)	98.45±29.72	78.14±25.60
9.	Mean Urinary Calcium/ Creatinine Ratio	0.04±0.02	0.12±0.05

TABLE 10: Mean±SD and the significant Difference in the Mean Urinary Calcium Levels between the Preeclamptic and the Control Groups

Group	Urinary Calcium Level (Mean±SD)	p-value	Inference
Preeclamptics	4.56±1.19	<0.0001	Difference is Statistically extremely significant
Control	9.23±3.49		

The Mean Urinary Calcium level was significantly lower in Preeclamptic women (4.56±1.19 mg/dL) than normotensive women (9.23±3.49 mg/dL) (p-value<0.0001).

TABLE 11: Mean±SD and the significant difference in the Mean Urinary Creatinine levels between the Preeclamptic and the Control groups

Group	Mean Urinary Creatinine levels (Mean±SD)	p-value	Inference
Preeclamptics	98.45±29.72	=0.0104	Difference is Statistically significant
Control	78.14±25.60		

Women destined to develop Preeclampsia had significant higher Mean Urinary Creatinine levels (98.45±29.72mg/dL) as compared to women who remained normotensive (78.14±25.60mg/dL) (p-value=0.0104).

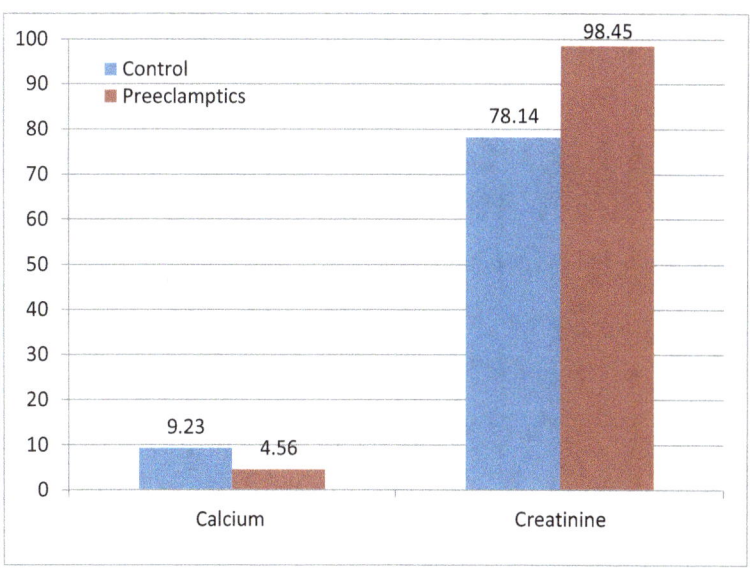

Figure 7: Bar chart showing Means Urinary Calcium and Creatinine levels in the Preeclamptic and the control groups

TABLE 12: Mean±SD and the significant difference in the Mean Urinary Calcium/Creatinine values in the Preeclamptics and the Control groups

Group	Urinary Calcium/Creatinine levels (Mean±SD)	p-value	Inference
Preeclamptics	0.04±0.02	<0.0001	Difference is Statistically extremely significant
Control	0.12±0.05		

As represented in TABLE: 12, the Mean Urinary Calcium/Creatinine level in Preeclamptic women was 0.04±0.02 and in the Control group, it was 0.12±0.05.

From the above table it is seen that there was a significant decrease in the Urinary Calcium/Creatinine Ratio in Preeclamptic cases when compared to the normal healthy women taken as Controls (p<0.0001).

TABLE 13: Association of Urinary Calcium/Creatinine Ratio with Preeclampsia

Calcium/ Creatinine Ratio	Preeclamptics (N %)	Normotensives (N %)	Test Result (N %)
Test positive (≤0.04)	10 (83.3%) (True positive)	2 (16.7%) (False positive)	12 (12%)
Test negative (> 0.04)	3 (3.4%) (False negative)	85 (96.6%) (True negative)	88 (88%)
Total cases	13	87	100

Above table shows the relationship of Urinary Calcium/Creatinine Ratio and development of Preeclampsia. Out of total 100 women 12 had Urinary Calcium/Creatinine Ratio ≤ 0.04 and amongst these 10 (83.3%) women had developed Preeclampsia later on. On the contrary, out of 88 women with Urinary Calcium/Creatinine Ratio >0.04 only 3 (3.4%) had Preeclampsia; while 85 (96.6%) women were remained normotensive.

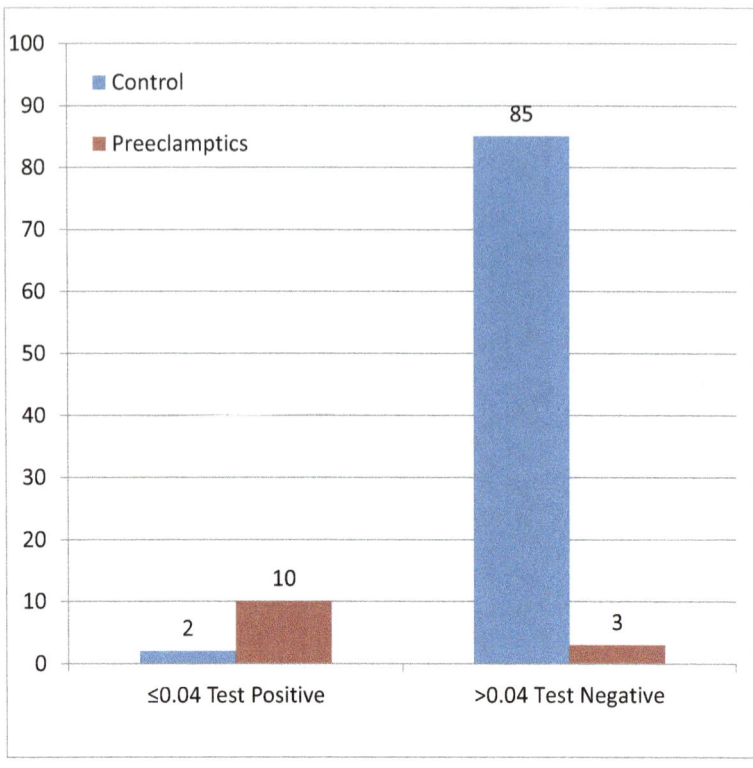

Figure 8: Bar chart shows the levels of Urinary Calcium/Creatinine Ratio in preeclamptics and control groups.

The above bar chart shows that there is a significant decrease in the Mean Urinary Calcium/Creatinine Ratio levels in Preeclamptic cases when compared to the normal healthy pregnant women taken as Controls.

TABLE 14: Validity of Urinary Calcium/Creatinine Ratio as predictor of Preeclampsia (results of Statistical analysis)

	Sensitivity	Specificity	PPV	NPV
Ca/Cr Ratio	76.90%	97.70%	83.33%	96.60%

Ca/Cr Ratio – Calcium/Creatinine Ratio; **PPV** - Positive Predictive Value; **NPV** - Negative Predictive Value.

Statistical analysis showed; when Urinary Calcium/Creatinine Ratio alone was taken as high risk factor for prediction of Preeclampsia; it was found to be highly significant (p<0.001); with Sensitivity 76.9%, Specificity 97.7%, Positive predictive value 83.33%, Negative predictive value 96.6% and Diagnostic accuracy 95%.

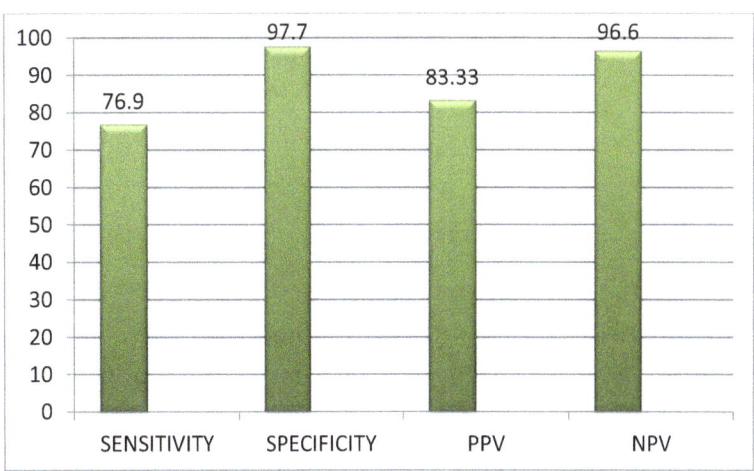

Figure 9: Bar chart showing results of Statistical analysis

SERUM LEVELS OF CALCIUM, MAGNESIUM AND URIC ACID IN PREECLAMPTIC WOMEN IN THIRD TRIMESTER IN COMPARISON WITH NORMAL PREGNANT WOMEN TAKEN AS CONTROLS:

The results from many clinical studies show the relationship between the aggravation of the hypertensive complication and the change in concentrations of various chemicals in mother's serum. Interestingly, variable Serum Calcium, Magnesium and Uric acid levels are found in Preeclamptic mothers.

TABLE 15: Age wise distribution of Preeclamptics and Control groups

Age (years)	Preeclamptic group	Control group
20-24	56	49
25-29	44	50
30-35	00	01
Total	100	100
Mean age	24.18	24.5

The Mean age in the Preeclamptic group and Control group were 24.18 years and 24.5 years respectively. In the Preeclamptic group 56% and in the Control group 49% belonged to the age between 20-24 years. In the Preeclamptic group 44% and in the Control group 50% belonged to the age between 25-29 years. In the Preeclamptic group 1% and in the Control group none belonged to age group of 30-35 years.

TABLE 16: Parity distribution in the Preeclamptics and Control groups

Gravidae	Cases	Controls	Total
Primigravidae	51 (51%)	54 (54%)	105
Multigravidae	49 (49%)	46 (46%)	95
Total	100	100	200

As represented in the table 16; amongst the Preeclamptic cases, the number of primigravidae was 51 and multigravidae was 49. The Control group included 54 primigravidae and 46 multiparous women. The cases and Controls were also matched with respect to parity (p-value =0.49 which is >0.05).

The above results show that the incidence of Preeclampsia was highest in primigravidae when compared to multiparous women.

Blood pressure:

The systolic blood pressure and diastolic blood pressure was measured using sphygmomanometer in the women left arm.

The values of systolic blood pressure and diastolic blood pressure and their standard deviation are presented in TABLE 17 for all the Preeclamptic groups.

TABLE 17: Mean and Standard deviation of Blood pressure in Preeclamptics and Control groups

Group	Mean Systolic blood pressure (mm Hg) with SD	Mean Diastolic blood pressure (mm Hg) with SD
Preeclamptics	145.32±6.66	96.8±5.00
Control	120.1±7.54	77.1±5.03
p-value	<0.0001	<0.0001

The Mean systolic blood pressure and diastolic blood pressure for Preeclamptic women were 145.32±6.66 mmHg and 96.80±5.00 mmHg respectively. For the Control group Systolic BP was 120.10±7.54 mm Hg and Diastolic BP was 77.10±5.03 mm Hg.

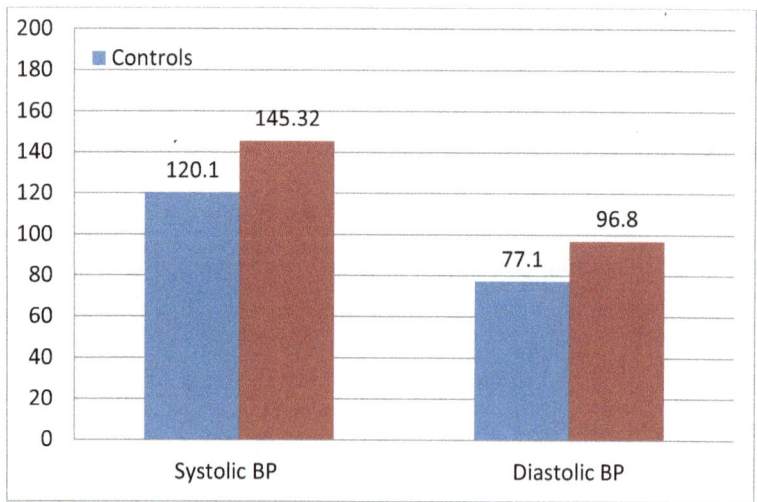

Figure 10: Bar diagram showing Mean Systolic BP and Diastolic BP (mm of Hg) in the Study

The above results show that in cases with Preeclampsia, the Systolic BP (p-value <0.0001) and Diastolic BP (p-value <0.0001) values were significantly higher in the cases when compared with the Control group.

SERUM CALCIUM

TABLE 18: Showing Mean±SD and the significant difference in the Mean Serum Calcium (mg/dL) between Preeclamptics and Control groups

Group	Serum Calcium (mg/dL) Mean±SD	p-value	Inference
Preeclamptics	8.27±0.37	<0.0001	Difference is extremely statistically significant
Control	9.06±0.27		

As represented in the TABLE 18, the Mean Serum Calcium in Preeclampsia was 8.27±0.37mg/dL and in Controls it was 9.06±0.27mg/dL. From this table it can be inferred that there is a significant decrease in Mean Serum Calcium values in Preeclamptic women when compared with normal healthy pregnant women (p<0.0001).

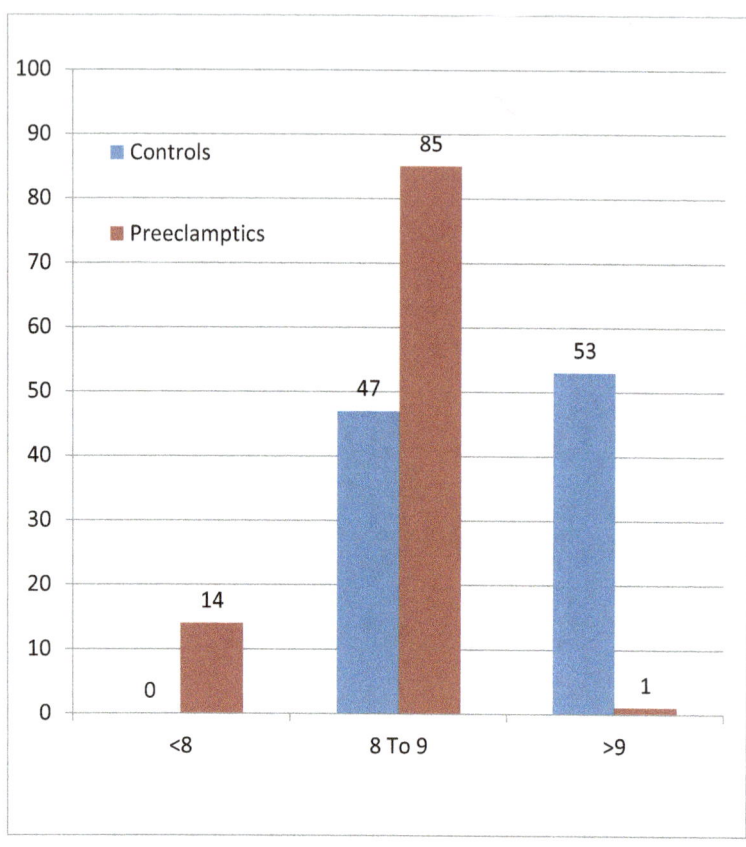

FIGURE 11: Bar chart showing the Mean Calcium levels (mg/dL) in the Preeclamptic and Control groups

The above bar chart shows that there is significant decrease in the Mean Calcium levels in Preeclamptic cases when compared with normal healthy pregnant women i.e., Controls.

SERUM MAGNESIUM:

TABLE 19: Showing Mean±SD and the significant difference in the Mean Serum Magnesium (mEq/L) between the Preeclamptic and Control groups

Group	Serum Magnesium (mEq/L)Mean±SD	p-value	Inference
Preeclamptics	1.99±0.13	=0.0308	Difference is Statistically significant.
Control	2.03±0.13		

Data are shown as Mean±SD; p-value were determined with student's t-test

As represented in table No. 19 the Mean Serum Magnesium levels in Preeclamptic women was 1.99±0.13 (mEq/L), and in the Control group it was 2.03±0.13 (mEq/L).

Thus it can be seen from the above table that there was statistically significant decrease in the Mean Magnesium levels in Preeclamptic cases when compared to the normal healthy pregnant women (p-value=0.0308 i.e. <0.05).

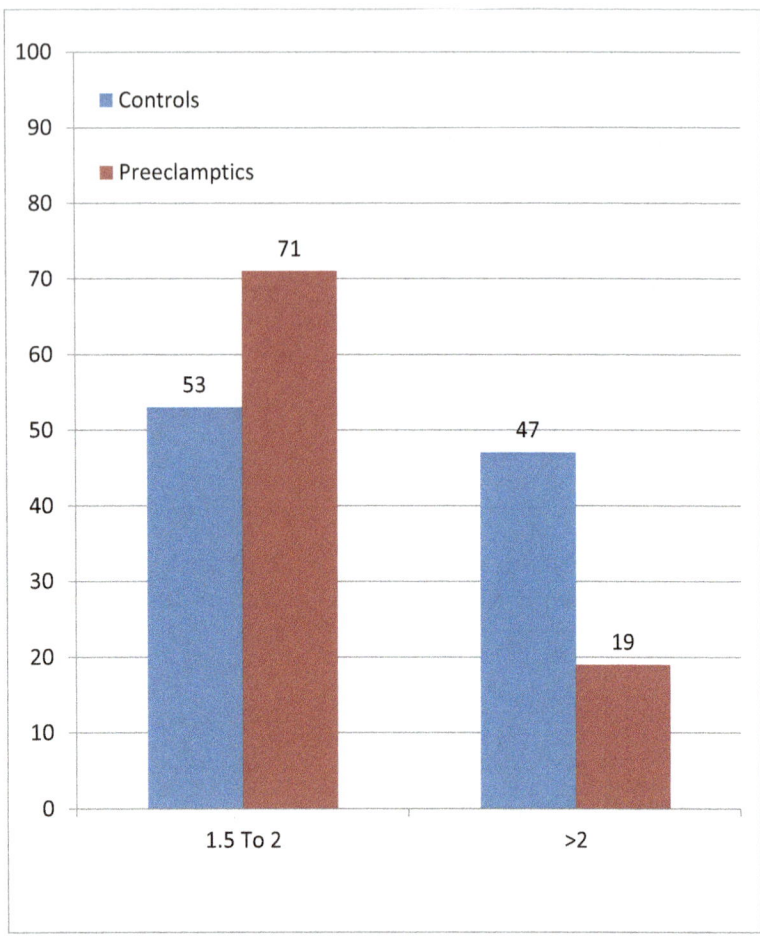

FIGURE 12: Bar chart showing the mean Serum Magnesium levels (mEq/L) in the Preeclamptic and Control groups

The above bar chart shows that there is a significant decrease in the Mean Magnesium levels in Preeclamptic cases when compared to the Control group.

SERUM URIC ACID:

TABLE 20: Showing Mean±SD and the significant difference in the Mean Serum Uric acid levels (mg/dL) between the Preeclamptic and Control groups

Group	Serum Uric-acid (mg/dL) Mean±SD	p-value	Inference
Preeclamptics	7.45±0.4	<0.0001	Difference is extremely statistically significant
Control	4.6±1.02		

As represented in table 20, the Mean Serum Uric acid level in Preeclamptic cases was 7.45±0.4mg/dL and in the Control group it was 4.6±1.02mg/dL.

The above table shows that there was extremely statistically significant increase in the Mean Uric acid levels in Preeclamptic cases when compared to the normal healthy pregnant women taken as Controls (p-value<0.0001).

Data in all the above concerning tables are shown as Mean±SD; p-value was determined with student's t-test.

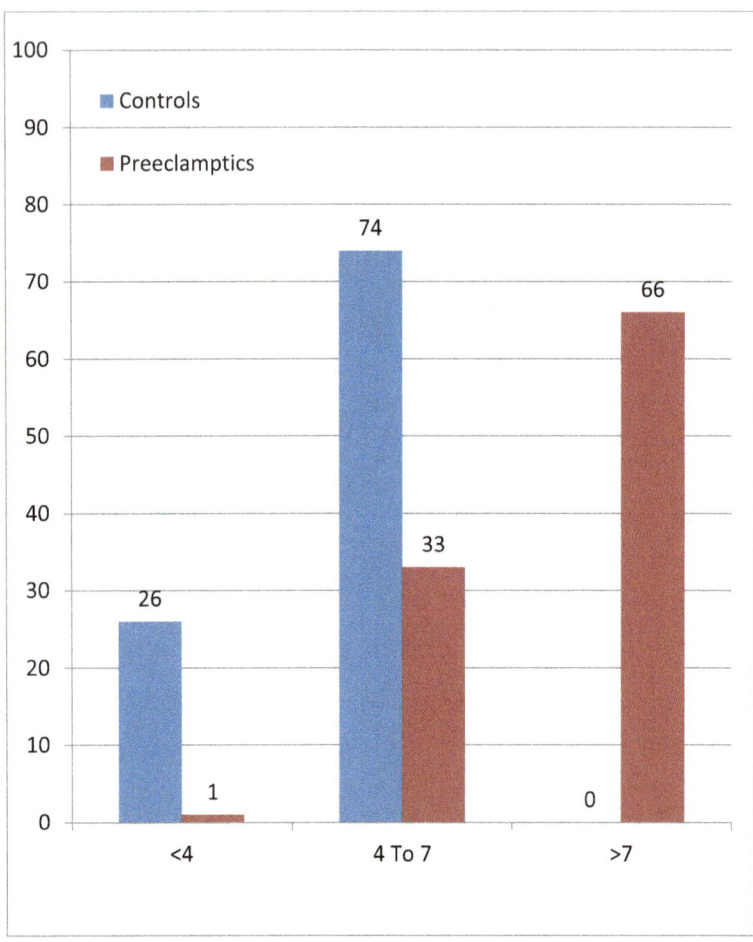

FIGURE 13: Bar chart shows the Mean Serum Uric acid levels (mg/dL) in the Preeclamptic and Control groups

The above bar chart shows that there is a significant increase in the Mean Serum Uric acid levels in Preeclamptic cases when compared to the normal healthy women.

DISCUSSION

When pregnancy is superimposed, on abnormal maternal medical conditions the metabolic milieu may be altered adversely for the fetus.

Preeclampsia diagnosed by increased blood pressure and de novo proteinuria, is a pregnancy specific disease associated with a high incidence of maternal and fetal morbidity and mortality. Despite intensive research and improved technology in recent decades the cause and pathophysiology of the syndrome remains enigmatic. Therefore its treatment is empirical and controversial[124]. The challenge of any screening test for Preeclampsia is to differentiate between those who are and will remain normotensive versus those who appear normal but will develop Preeclampsia.

STUDY: TO DETERMINE THE PREDICTIVE VALUE OF CALCIUM TO CREATININE RATIO IN ASYMPTOMATIC NORMOTENSIVE PREGNANT WOMEN IN SECOND TRIMESTER

Many scientists have done a lot of research on these lines. Our work had progressed in the same direction on the guide lines laid by these scientists.

In our study, we have assessed the relationship between hypocalciuria and Preeclampsia; measured by Urinary Calcium/Creatinine Ratio. Study was done in 100 asymptomatic, normotensive pregnant women between 20-28 weeks gestation (**For estimation of Urinary Calcium/Creatinine Ratio**). Out of 100 women, who were followed from 20-28 weeks of gestation till delivery, **Group-B** developed Preeclampsia - 13 (incidence 13%) whereas **Group-A** - 87 (87%) remained normotensive.

In present study, we found that 53.84% of cases belonged to **age group** between 20-24 years and 38% belonged to 25-29 years. This is in accordance with risk factors of Preeclampsia listed in text book of Obstetrics by **D.C. Dutta** (2004); which states that Preeclampsia occurs more commonly in early young aged primigravidae[125]. Also it is started in risk factors of Preeclampsia mentioned in Danforth's text book of Obstetrics and Gynecology (2008)[126].

URINARY CALCIUM:

In the present study, we found that the mean Urinary Calcium levels in spot urine sample of control and preeclamptic groups were 9.23±3.49mg/dL and 4.56±1.19mg/dL respectively. It was lesser in preeclamptic group as compared to the control group. And in a same way; **Taufield et al** (1987) found a significantly lower mean Urinary Calcium level in women with Preeclampsia than in normotensive women[94]. The mean Urinary Calcium levels were reported lesser in preeclamptic women **by Kazemi AFN et al** (2010) [101].

URINARY CREATININE:

In our study, we also found that the mean Urinary Creatinine levels in spot urine samples of control and preeclamptic groups were 78.14±25.60mg/dL and 98.45±29.72mg/dL respectively. It was higher in preeclamptic group as compared to the control group. And in the same way it was also reported higher in preeclamptic women (110.61±11.53) as compared to the control group (109.15±56.42) by **Kazemi AFN et al** (2010)[101].

URINARY CALCIUM/CREATININE RATIO:

In the study of **Rodriguez MH et al** (1988), 83% pregnant women with low Calcium/Creatinine Ratio developed Preeclampsia[20]. In study of **Kamra et al** (1997) 71.4% pregnant women with low Calcium/Creatinine Ratio developed Preeclampsia[109]. In the study **of J Kar et al** (2002), 64.2% pregnant women with low Calcium/Creatinine Ratio developed Preeclampsia[104].

Huikeshoven FJM et al (1990) concluded that the measurement of Urinary Calcium excretion is of value for the study of pregnant women with Preeclampsia, both in terms of 24 hour excretion and in the Urinary Calcium/Creatinine Ratio of a single urine sample[95].

Raniolo E et al (1991) determined that the Urinary Calcium/Creatinine Ratio was not significantly different between the groups of normotensive pregnant women (0.52±0.32) and women with Preeclampsia (0.49±0.32). These findings don't correlate; what we have found during our study[108].

Suzuki Y et al (1992) studied 348 healthy women at 20 weeks of gestation and underwent urine analysis to determine their Calcium/Creatinine Ratio as a means to predict Preeclampsia in patients showing no symptoms. Out of them 249 remained healthy and 38 women developed Preeclampsia at the time of delivery. And they found that the Calcium/Creatinine Ratio was significantly lower in the women with Preeclampsia than in the healthy pregnant women, and it was especially low in those with Preeclampsia who had no family history of hypertension[103].

Ye Y et al (1995) in their study collected data of twenty four hour Urinary Calcium excretion and determined Urinary Calcium/ Creatinine Ratio in normal pregnant and preeclamptic women. They found that 24 hour Urinary Calcium excretion, Urinary Calcium concentration and Calcium/Creatinine Ratio in preeclamptic group were significantly lower than that in normal pregnant women (p-value< 0.01). 3 mmol/L of Urinary Calcium concentration and 0.04 of Calcium/Creatinine Ratio were chosen as predictive thresholds for development of Preeclampsia, with sensitivity of 76.2%, 81.0% and specificity of 97.5%, 98.2% respectively. These findings are very much similar to our study. This confirms that Urinary Calcium/Creatinine Ratio is significantly lower in preeclamptic women than normal pregnant women no matter urine is collected for whole 24 hours or spot as was in our study[102].

Ozcan T et al (1995) who investigated the predictive value of decreasing Calcium to creatinine ratio in a spot urine sample reported that it might be an effective marker for Preeclampsia[99]. Saudan PJ et al (1998) have reported a sensitivity of only 68% and specificity of 70% [98] and Izumi A et al (1997) found that it had limited value in prediction of

Preeclampsia, but the threshold value used was 0.10 by the former and Izumi et al carried out the test in early pregnancy, at less than or equal to 12 weeks of gestation[127]. Kazerooni T et al (2003) evaluating between 20-24 weeks of gestation[97] and Kar J et al (2002) evaluating the predictive value of Calcium/Creatinine Ratio at less than or equal to 0.04 between 20-34 weeks of gestation (similar to our study), have reported that it was a satisfactory test for prediction of Preeclampsia and could be an effective method for screening asymptomatic women for Preeclampsia[104].

Sheela CN et al (2011) in their study found that Calcium/Creatinine Ratio in a spot urine sample was less than or equal to 0.04 had a sensitivity of 69.20%, specificity of 98.20% with a PPV and NPV of 85.70% and 95.80% respectively. This confirms that there is a definite relationship between low Urinary Calcium/Creatinine Ratio and development of Preeclampsia[36].

In a similar way we have found Calcium/Creatinine Ratio from spot urine samples between 20-28 weeks of gestation was less than or equal to 0.04 had a sensitivity of 76.90%, specificity of 97.70% with a good Positive predictive value and Negative predictive value of 83.33% and 96.60% respectively. So, it was statistically appropriate test for prediction of Preeclampsia.

TABLE 21: Comparative study of Urinary Calcium/Creatinine Ratio in different research papers

Author (year)	Preeclamptic women	Normal Pregnant women (Control)
Huikeshoven et al[95] (1990)	0.03±0.03	0.44±0.32
Frenkel et al[128] (1991)	0.049±0.03	0.23±0.17
Raniolo et al[108] (1993)	0.049±0.32	0.52±0.32
Ozcan et al[99] (1995)	0.047±0.026	0.1466±0.1353
Suarez et al[96] (1996)	0.23 (0.14–0.32) *	0.29 (0.26–0.32) *
Kazerooni et al[97] (2003)	0.306±0.27	0.52±0.3
Smith-Adije et al[129] (2006)	0.2±0.2	0.6±0.4
Mandira et al[130] (2008)	0.12±0.11	0.21±0.10
Mc Growder et al[107] (2009)	0.17±0.03	0.45±0.08
Gasnier et al[131] (2011)	SPE 0.0108 (0–0.14) * MPE 0.05 (0.01–0.36) *	0.0995 (0.04–0.23) *
Present study (2013)	0.04±0.02	0.12±0.05

*Data has been expressed as mean±standard deviation for symmetrical distribution and median (minimum-maximum) for asymmetrical distribution. All the values above were significant. SPE – Severe Preeclampsia and MPE – Mild Preeclampsia.

The following table shows six studies that have investigated the predictive value of low Calcium/Creatinine Ratio in Preeclampsia.

TABLE 22: Comparison of predictive value of Urinary Calcium/ Creatinine ratio in present study with other studies

Author & Year	No. of patients	Sensitivity %	Specificity %	PPV %	NPV %
Rodriguez et al[20] (1988)	88	70	95	64	96
Ramos SL et al[28] (1991)	99	88	84	32	99
Ritu Kamra et al[109] (1994)	104	71.40	95.50	71.40	95.50
Ozcan et al[99] (1995)	56	63	96	71	93
J Kar et al[104] (1999)	100	75	94.38	64.23	96.51
Sheela CN et al[36] (2011)	200	69.20	98.20	85.70	95.50
Present study (2013)	100	76.90	97.70	83.33	96.60

In all the above studies it was observed that patients who subsequently developed Preeclampsia had low Urinary Calcium excretion. Majority of the patient developed Preeclampsia were found to have Calcium/Creatinine Ratio of less than 0.04.

STUDY: THE AIM OF THIS STUDY WAS TO MEASURE SERUM LEVELS OF CALCIUM, MAGNESIUM AND URIC ACID IN PREECLAMPTIC WOMEN AND TO COMPARE THOSE WITH NORMAL PREGNANT WOMEN IN THIRD TRIMESTER

We also collected data for estimation of Serum Calcium, Serum Magnesium and Serum Uric acid from 100 pregnant women with diagnosis of Preeclampsia in the third trimester (**Group-II**) and 100 normal, age matched pregnant women in the third trimester (**Group–III**) as Control for Group–II; that admitted in the Department of Obstetrics and Gynecology for parturition.

SERUM CALCIUM:

In present study, we found that 56% of cases belonged to **age group** between 20-24 years and 44% belonged to 25-29 years. This is in accordance with risk factors of Preeclampsia listed in text book of Obstetrics by **D.C. Dutta** (2004); which states that Preeclampsia occurs more commonly in early young aged primigravidae[125]. Also it is started in risk factors of Preeclampsia mentioned in **Danforth's** text book of Obstetrics and Gynecology (2008)[126].

Also we found Preeclampsia was more common in **primigravidae** (51%) than multigravidae (49%), that more common in young primigravidae. The same is mentioned in the text book of Obstetrics by **D.C. Dutta** (2004), that Preeclampsia is seen more commonly in young primigravidae (70%)[125] and in **Danforth's** text book of Obstetrics and Gynecology (2008), which it occurs more commonly in nulliparous women of extremes of ages[126].

In our study the mean Serum Calcium levels in preeclamptic group and in control group were 8.27±0.37 mg/dL and 9.06±0.27mg/dL respectively.

Our findings are comparable with **Malas NO et al** (2001) who have also observed decreased Serum Calcium levels in preeclamptic women when compared to the control group[113]. **Sukonpan K et al** (2005) in their study also observed that mean Serum Calcium concentration in preeclamptic pregnant women is significantly lower than that in normal pregnant women (9.0±0.4 mg/dL vs. 9.7±0.7 mg/dL, p-value<0.0001)[6]. **Chaurasia PP** (2012) observed that the Serum Calcium in preeclamptic women and in normal pregnant were 8.9±0.4 mg/dL vs. 9.7±0.7 mg/dL, p-value<0.0001 respectively, significantly lower than that in normal pregnant women[29].

Chanvitya P et al (2008) found that the Serum Calcium in severe preeclamptic women was significantly lower (8.7 ± 0.59 mg/dL vs. 8.99±0.31 mg/dL, p-value= 0.045; and 9.05±0.52 mg/dL, p-value= 0.014) than in normal pregnant women and mild preeclamptic women respectively, but there was no difference between normal and mild preeclamptic women. Similarly we also found that Serum Calcium levels were lesser in **Group-II** (i.e. preeclamptic women) than in **Group-III** (i.e. Normotensive women)[30].

Roodsari V et al (2008) in a case-control study in 50 preeclamptic and 50 normal pregnant women found that Calcium levels had no significant differences (9.16±0.75mg/dL vs. 9.47±1.58 mg/dL) in preeclamptic and normal pregnant women. In contrast to this study, our results favors that there is a definitive correlation between low Serum Calcium levels with development of Preeclampsia[7].

Alavi A et al (2012) have done a cross-sectional study in 100 healthy and 48 hypertensive pregnant women with singleton pregnancy who were at ≥ 28 weeks of gestation were included and Serum Calcium levels were compared between these three groups. Hypertensive group consisted of 28 subjects with mild Preeclampsia, 17 with severe Preeclampsia and 3 were found to be Eclamptic. Mean Serum Calcium level was 7.88±0.94 mg/dL in mild preeclamptics, 6.28±4.50 in severe preeclamptics and 5.04U±4.60 in Eclamptics Vs. 8.28±0.77 mg/dL in control group. Thus it concluded that mean Serum Calcium level was significantly lowers in hypertensive pregnant women than healthy pregnant women which matches the findings of our study[111].

Sayyed AK et al (2013) have conducted the study in subjects aged between 18-35 years comprised of three groups: **Group-I** preeclamptic women, **Group-II** Normal pregnant women, **Group-III** Normal healthy controls. Serum was analyzed for estimation of Calcium. The results showed that Serum Calcium levels were significantly decreased (p-value<0.01) in preeclamptics as compared to normal pregnant women as well as healthy controls. Hypocalcaemia seen in the preeclamptic women may be responsible for the vascular pathology associated with onset of Preeclampsia. Hence adjuvant supplementation of Calcium may prevent further progression of Preeclampsia[117].

Sendhav S et al (2013) in their cross sectional case control study conducted with 90 subjects found that there were significantly low Serum Calcium levels in severe preeclamptic women as compared to normal pregnant and mild preeclamptic women. Also there was no significant difference found between normal and mild preeclamptic women[118].

The above findings show that hypocalcaemia could be a risk factor for the development of Preeclampsia. This data support the hypothesis that Calcium might be a cause in the development of Preeclampsia. The effect of Serum Calcium and its correlation with change in blood pressure could be explained by the level of intracellular concentration of Calcium. When Serum Calcium concentration decreases; there is an increase of intracellular Calcium concentration; which leads to the constriction of smooth muscles in blood vessels and also increases in vascular resistance.

SERUM MAGNESIUM:

In the present study, the mean Serum Magnesium levels in cases of Preeclampsia were 1.99±0.13 mEq/L and in controls it was 2.03±0.13 mEq/L. There was significant decrease in the Serum levels of Magnesium in preeclamptic cases when compared with the control group.

However, **Sukonpan K et al** (2005) have observed that Serum Magnesium concentration in preeclamptic women is significantly lower than that in normal pregnant women (0.77±0.08 mmol/L vs. 0.85±0.09 mmol/L, p-value=0.001)[6].

Roodsari V et al (2008) in a case-control study showed that Serum Magnesium levels in the preeclamptic women were significantly lower than those of individuals with normal pregnancy (1.92±0.37 mg/dL vs. 2.29±0.69 mg/dL), (p-value<0.01)[7].

Chanvitya P et al (2008) found that there was no difference in Serum Magnesium among normal pregnancy and both groups of Preeclampsia[30]. Similarly **Golmohammed LS et al** (2008) have found no significant decrease in Serum Magnesium levels in preeclamptic cases when compared to the control group[31].

Chaurasia PP (2012) observed that the Serum Magnesium concentration in preeclamptic women (0.75±0.08 mmol/L) was significantly lower than that of normal pregnant women (0.85±0.09 mmol/L)[29].

Sayyed AK et al (2013) have conducted the study into three groups. They found the Serum Magnesium levels in **Group – I** i.e.: preeclamptic women (1.28±1.08 mg/dL), in **Group – II** i.e.: pregnant women of same gestational age (1.80±0.47 mg/dL) and in **Group – III** i.e.: normal healthy controls (2.31±0.35 mg/dL). Serum Magnesium levels were significantly lower in **Group – I** (p-value< 0.001) when compared with **Group – II** & **Group – III**[112].

Sendhav S et al (2013) in their cross sectional case control study found that there were significantly low Serum Magnesium levels in severe preeclamptic women (1.64±0.35mg/dL) as compared to normal pregnant (2.12±0.17mg/dL) and mild preeclamptic women (2.17±0.18mg/dL). Also there was no significant difference found between normal and mild preeclamptic women[118].

Generally, the hypomagnesaemia in most pregnant women is associated with hemodilution, altered renal clearance and consumption of minerals by the growing fetus. Magnesium is essential cofactor for enzymes and plays an important role in neurochemical transmission and peripheral vasodilatation.

This study showed that both Serum Calcium and Serum Magnesium levels in preeclamptic pregnant women are lower than in normal pregnant women. This study supports the hypothesis that hypocalcaemia and hypomagnesaemia are possible etiologies of Preeclampsia.

SERUM URIC ACID:

The association between Serum Uric acid and Preeclampsia has been investigated in many studies. In the present study the mean Serum Uric acid in cases of Preeclampsia was 7.45±0.40 mg/dL and in controls it was 4.60±1.02 mg/dL. There was an extremely statistically significant increase in Uric acid levels in preeclamptic group compared to the control group.

Almasganj F et al (2004) observed that Serum Uric acid levels were higher in hypertensive pregnant women as compared with healthy pregnant women[132]. And **Roberts JM et al** (2005) have shown the increase in Serum Uric acid level with the severity of Preeclampsia[46]. Also **Taner C et al** (2004) agrees with our findings where Serum Uric acid levels are elevated in preeclamptic patients when compared to the controls[133].

Our findings agree with the study done by **Chanvitya P et al** (2008), who have shown that hyperuricemia may induce hypertension and vascular disease. The Serum Uric acid in severe preeclamptic women was significantly more than normal pregnant women and mild preeclamptic women (7.01±1.93 mg/dL vs. 5.33±1.23 mg/dL, p-value<0.001; and 5.95±1.9 mg/dL, p-value=0.044 respectively). There was no significant difference in Serum Uric acid between normal pregnant women and mild preeclamptic women[30].

Alavi A et al (2012) in their study found that mean Serum Uric acid level was 5.32±1.41 mg/dL in hypertensive pregnant women and 4.55±1.14 mg/dL in control group i.e.: healthy pregnant women (p-value=0.001)[111].

Sendhav S et al (2013) in their cross sectional case control study found that there were significantly high Serum Uric acid levels in severe preeclamptic women as compared to normal pregnant and mild preeclamptic women. Also there was no significant difference found between normal and mild preeclamptic women[118].

Hyperuricemia is believed to result from decreased renal excretion as a consequence of Preeclampsia, also results from increased production secondary to tissue ischemia and oxidative stress. Hyperuricemia induces endothelial dysfunction and may induce hypertension and vascular disease.

Renal excretion of Calcium and Phosphate increases during pregnancy. Excretion usually increases during each trimester, with maximum levels reached during the third trimester. Proteinuria and alterations of phosphate and most notably Calcium excretion are common findings of hypertension and some renal disorders in general. There is a decrease in Urinary Calcium levels in Preeclampsia. Our findings in Preeclampsia agree with the results of **Sanchez-Ramos** (1991)[26] and **Taufield** (1987)[94]. The reason for hypercalciuria in pregnancy is probably the increased glomerular filtration rate. Because parathyroid hormone and calcitonin levels were not altered in the patients with Preeclampsia, it was concluded that the differences in Calcium metabolism were not related to alterations in the secretion of these hormones.

The above findings show that alteration in Calcium, Magnesium and Uric acid metabolism during pregnancy could be one of the potential causes of Preeclampsia.

SUMMARY AND CONCLUSION

Preeclampsia is idiopathic multisystem disorder specific to human pregnancy. Hypertension is a universal problem; and it complicates at least 10% of all the pregnancies[2].

The present study was done for early prediction of Preeclampsia. Early prediction of this disease would help in reducing maternal and fetal morbidity and mortality.

The study was conducted in the Department of Biochemistry in collaboration with Department of Obstetrics and Gynecology, Sri Aurobindo Medical College & Post Graduate Institute, Indore during the period January 2012 to January 2013. 100 Normotensive, asymptomatic pregnant women **(Group–I)** were registered between 20-28 weeks of pregnancy with no history of hypertension, renal disease or diabetes. Spot urine sample was collected for estimation of Urinary Calcium/Creatinine Ratio. All subjects were followed up till delivery and then grouped in to **preeclamptic (B)** and normal healthy pregnant women i.e. **control (A)**.

Our study had shown Urinary Calcium/Creatinine Ratio ≤0.04 proved to be the predictor of subsequent development of Preeclampsia. In this study, we found the Positive predictive value of Urinary Calcium/Creatinine Ratio - 83.33%, Negative predictive value - 96.60%, Sensitivity -76.90%, Specificity -97.70% and Diagnostic accuracy -95%.

Various precipitating factors such as Calcium, Magnesium, Uric acid and Proteinuria have been implicated in the etiology and severity of Preeclampsia and its manifestation.

Therefore, in the present study; we have also studied the role of Serum Calcium, Magnesium and Uric acid as possible etiological factors in Preeclampsia.

Interestingly, the significant reduction in serum Calcium and Magnesium are found in preeclamptic women in our study and agrees with the physiological role of both Calcium and Magnesium in humans[7].

In **Group-II,** 100 women with Preeclampsia and in **Group-III,** 100 normal healthy pregnant women as Controls were selected for the study. There was decrease in Serum Calcium and Magnesium levels and increase in Serum Uric acid levels in preeclamptic women when compared with normal healthy pregnant women taken as Controls. The changes in Serum Calcium, Magnesium and Uric acid levels were statistically significant.

However, the present study showed Hypocalcaemia, Hypomagnesaemia and Hyperuricemia in Preeclampsia; suggesting the role of Calcium, Magnesium and Uric acid in the etiology of Preeclampsia.

Constant monitoring of Serum Calcium, Magnesium and Uric acid; hence may reduce severity and complications of Preeclampsia and improve fetal outcome by early treatment.

CONCLUSIONS

Preeclampsia is a multifaceted disorder related to pregnancy. In order to assess the predictive value of different biomarkers related to it; and finally proposing the best marker for routine use in clinical settings for its screening; this study has been undertaken.

Screening, the deliberate examination of substantial segments of the population in search for disease at its earliest stages, is a logical extension of the role of preventive medicine and one that is becoming increasingly popular. Ideally a screening test should be inexpensive, easy to perform, readily interpretable and readily available to the entire population at risk. Also a screening test for the entire population must be acceptable to the population.

Ongoing research shows abundant evidence that the pathophysiological changes of Preeclampsia were present long before the clinical presentation of the disorder, which probably explains why all the management of Preeclampsia are only palliative till delivery. This indicates that for an effective therapy to be successful, the therapy has to be instituted before clinically evident disease.

The study can be concluded as follows:

- In the present study the Urinary Calcium/Creatinine Ratio in asymptomatic normotensive pregnant women in second trimester had been measured and followed them up to the delivery. The statistical analysis of the results showed that there lies a very significant relationship between low Urinary Calcium/Creatinine Ratio and the development of Preeclampsia later in pregnancy.

- In the present study the Serum levels of Calcium, Magnesium and Uric acid in preeclamptic women had been measured and compared those with normal pregnant women in third trimester. Based on the results of the present study and data available from literature, it is clear that in Preeclampsia, the Serum levels of Calcium and Magnesium were found lower than normal while Serum Uric acid levels were higher indicating the possible role of these biomarkers in the pathophysiological of Preeclampsia.

- We have developed a predictive model for **screening Preeclampsia** and subgroups at *increased risk* in which prior therapy might be indicated **to prevent maternal and perinatal morbidity and mortality**.

Thus predictors of Preeclampsia with high sensitivity and moderate specificity will be useful initially in the conduct of clinical trials and perhaps eventually for therapy in future.

Spot Urinary Calcium/Creatinine Ratio is simple, cheap and easy to perform, noninvasive, specific and sensitive; which could also add up the diagnostic predictability of Preeclampsia. The role of Calcium/ Creatinine Ratio appears to be significant & it may be used as additional marker for Preeclampsia in Antenatal care (ANC) profile. Therefore, we recommend that analysis of spot Urinary Calcium/Creatinine Ratio may be an effective screening method for impending Preeclampsia and useful to identify population at greater risk. So, it could be included in **primary prevention programs**.

Serum Calcium, Magnesium and Uric acid levels should also be estimated as a part of **Secondary prevention programs** in diagnosed cases of Preeclampsia to prevent further complications.

Laboratory facilities should be developed at Primary health centre level for Spot urine examination for above mentioned markers to prevent disease and its comorbidities.

REFERENCES

1. Freinkel N. Effects of the conceptus on maternal metabolism during pregnancy. Leibel BS, Wrenshall GA, Edn. On the Nature and Treatment of Diabetes, Amsterdam: *Excerpta Medica*; 1965:679-688.

2. Indumati K, Kodliwadmath MV and Sheela MK. The Role of serum electrolytes in Pregnancy induced hypertension. *Journal of Clinical and Diagnostic Research* 2011; **5**(1):66-69.

3. Redman CWG and Jefferis M. Revised definition of preeclampsia. *Lancet* 1988; **1**:809–812.

4. Pridjan G and Puschett JB. Preeclampsia Part-1 clinical and pathophysiologic considerations. *Obstet Gynecol Surv* 2002; **57**:598–618.

5. Walker JJ. Preclampsia. *Lancet* 2000; **356**:260-1265.

6. Sukonpan K and Phupong V. Serum calcium and serum magnesium in normal and preeclamptic pregnancy. *Arch Gynecol Obstet* 2005; **273**: 12–16.

7. Roodsari V, Fatemeh and Ayati et al. Serum Calcium and Magnesium in Preeclamptic and Normal Pregnancies: A Comparative Study. *J Reprod Infertil* 2008; **9**(3):256-262.

8. Repke JT and Villar J. Pregnancy-induced hypertension and low birth weight: the role of calcium. *Am J Clin Nutr* 1991; **54**:237S–241S.

9. Barker P and Kingdom J. Preeclampsia. RCOG Press, Canada 1st Edn. 2004; 25-35.

10. Cunningham FG, Leveno KJ, Bloom SL, Hauth JC and Gilstrap LC et al. Williams Obstetrics. McGraw Hill, USA 22nd Edn. 2005.

11. O'Brien WF. The prediction of preeclampsia. *Clinical Obstetrics and Gynecology* 1992; **35**: 351-364.

12. Steel SA, Pearce JM, McParkland P and Chamberlain GVP. Early Doppler ultrasound screening in predicting of hypertensive disorders of pregnancy. *Lancet* 1990; **335**:1548-1550.

13. McParkland P, Pearce JM and Chamberlain GVP. Doppler ultrasound and aspirin: recognition and prevention of pregnancy induced hypertension. *Lancet* 1990; **335**:1552-1553.

14. Jacobson SL, Imhof R and Manning N. The value of Doppler assessment of the uteroplacental circulation in predicting preeclampsia or intrauterine growth retardation. *American Journal of Obstetrics and Gynecology* 1990; **162**:110-114.

15. Redman CW, Beilen LJ, Bonnar J and Wilkinson RH. Plasma-urate measurements in predicting fetal death in hypertensive pregnancy. *Lancet* 1976; **1**:1370-1372.

16. Gant NF, Chand S, Worley RJ and Daley GL. A clinical test useful for predicting the development of acute hypertension in pregnancy. *American Journal of Obstetrics and Gynecology* 1974; **120**:1-8.

17. Phelan JP, Everidge GL, Welder TL and Newman C. Is the supine test an adequate means of predicting acute hypertension in pregnancy? *American Journal of Obstetrics and Gynecology* 1977; **128**:173-176.

18. Ramos JG and Martins-Costa S. Teste da pressão supina. Revista Hospital de Clínicas de Porto Alegre 1989; **9**:125-127.

19. Gant NF, Daley GL, Chand S and Worley RJ. A study of angiotensin II pressor response throughout primigravid pregnancy. *Journal of Clinical Investigation* 1973; **52**:2682-2689.

20. Rodriguez MH, Masaki DI and Mestman J et al. Calcium/creatinine ratio and microalbuminuria in the prediction of preeclampsia. *Am J Obstet Gynecol* 1988 Dec; **159**(6):1452-5.

21. Erikson HO, Hansen PK, Brocks V and Jewsen BA. Plasma fibronectin concentration in pre-eclampsia. *Acta Obstetrica et Gynecologica Scandinavica* 1987; **66**:25-30.

22. Weiner CP and Brandt J. Plasma antithrombin III activity: an aid in the diagnosis of preeclampsia-eclampsia. *American Journal of Obstetrics and Gynecology* 1982; **142**: 275-277.

23. Halhali A, Diaz L, Avila E et al. Decreased fractional urinary calcium excretion and serum, 1,25- dihydroxyvitamin D and IGF-levels in preeclampsia. *J Steroid Biochem Mol Biol* 2007; **103**:803-6.

24. Szmidt-Adjide V, Vendittelli F, David S et al. Calciuria and preeclampsia: a case control study. *Eur J Obstet Gynecol Reprod Biol* 2006; **125**:193-8.

25. Segovia BL, Vega IT, Villarreal EC et al. Hypocalciuria during pregnancy as a risk factor of preeclampsia. *Ginecol Obstet Mex* 2004; **72**:570-4.

26. Ramos S, Sandeoni S, Andres FJ, Kauntiz AM. Calcium excretion in preeclampsia. *Obstet Gynaecol* 1991; **77**:510-513.

27. Suarez Ur, Trelles JG, Miyahira JM. Urinary calcium in asymptomatic primigravidas who later developed preeclampsia. *Obstet Gynaecol* 1996; **87**:79-82.

28. Ramos SL, David C, Jones, Cullen MT. Urinary calcium as an early marker for preeclampsia. *Obstet Gynaecol* 1991; **77**:685-688.

29. Chaurasia PP, Jadav PA, Jasani JH. Changes in serum calcium and Magnesium level in preeclampsia vs normal pregnancy. *International J of Biomedical and advance Research* 2012; **3**(6):511-513.

30. Chanvitya P, Boonsri K. Serum calcium, magnesium and uric acid in preeclampsia in normal pregnancy. *Journal of Medical Association Thailand* 2008; **91**(7):968-73.

31. Golmohmmad L S, Amirabi A et al. Evaluation of serum calcium, magnesium, copper and zinc levels in women with preeclampsia. *Iran Journal of Medical Sciences* 2008; **33**(4):231-234.

32. Skjaerven R, Wilcox A, Lie RT. The interval between pregnancies and the risk of preeclampsia. *N Engl J Med* 2002; **346**:33-8.

33. Kang DH, Finch J, Nakagawa T, Karumanchi SA, Kanellis J, Granger J, et al. Uric acid, endothelial dysfuction and preeclampsia: searching for a pathogenetic link. *J Hypertens* 2004; **22**:229-235.

34. Wilson JMG, Jungner G: Principles and Practice of Screening for Disease. In *Public Health* Geneva: *WHO* 1968; *Page No. 34.*

35. Audibert F. Screening for pre-eclampsia: the quest for the Holy Grail? Lancet 2005; **365**:1367-1369.

36. Sheela CN, Beena SR and Mhaskar A. Calcium-creatinine ratio and microalbuminuria in prediction of preeclampsia. *Journal of Obstetrics and Gynaecology of India* 2011; **61**(1):72-76.

37. Baha M, Sibai MD. Pitfalls in diagnosis and management of preeclampsia. *Am J Obstet and Gynecol* 1988; **159**(1):1-4.

38. Chesley LC. Hypertensive disorders of pregnancy. New York: Appleton – Century - Crofts, 1978.

39. Singh HJ. Pre-Eclampsia: Is it all in the placenta? *Malaysian Journal of Medical Sciences* 2009; **16**(1):7-15.

40. Hughes EC. Obstetric-Gynecologic terminology. *Philadelphia, Davis*, 1972; 422-423.

41. Davey DA, McGillvray I. The classification and definition of the hypertensive disorders of pregnancy. *Am J Obstet Gynecol* 1988; **158**:892-898.

42. National high blood pressure education program (NHBPEP) working group report on high blood pressure in pregnancy. *Am J Obstet Gynecol* 1990; **163**:1689-1712.

43. Cunningham FG, MacDonald PC, Grant NF, Levano KJ, Gilstrop LC. Hypertensive disorders in pregnancy. Williams Obstetrics, USA: prentice-Hall International Inc 19th edition 1993; 763-817.

44. American Congress of Obstetrics and Gynecology (ACOG) Practice Bulletin No. 29; July 2001:Reaffirmed 2010.

45. Roberts JM, Lain KY. Recent Insights into the pathogenesis of pre-eclampsia. *Placenta* 2002; **23**:359-72.

46. Roberts JM, Gammill HS. Preeclampsia: recent insights. Hypertension 2005; **46**:1243-9.

47. Chesley LC. *Obstet and Gynecol* 1985; **65**:423.

48. Zeek PM and Assali NS. Vascular changes in the desidua associated with eclamptogenic toxemia of pregnancy. *Am J Clin Path* 1950; **20**:1099-1109.

49. Lindheimer MD, Katz AI. The Kidney; Saunders, Philadelphia 3rd edn. 1986.

50. Boyd JD and Hamilton WJ. The human placenta. Heffer and Sons, Cambridge, England 1970.

51. Sibai BM, Schneider JM, Morrison JC et al. The late postpartum eclampsia controversy. *Obstet Gynecol* 1980; **55**:74-8.

52. Gary CF, Levena KJ, Bloom SL, Hauth JC, Gilstrap L, Wenstrom KD. Hypertensive disorders in pregnancy. In: Williams obstetrics. 22nd ed., New York; McGraw Hill, 2005. 761-808.

53. Dekker GA, Sibi BM. Etiology and pathogenesis of preeclampsia : current concepts. *Am J Obstet Gynecol*. 1998; **179**:1359-64.

54. Hayashi M, Hamada Y, Ohkura T. Elevation of granulocyte colony stimulating factor in the placenta and blood in pre-eclampsia. *Am J Obstet Gynecol*. 2005; **190**:456-60.

55. Gervasi MT, Chaiworapongsa T, Pacora P. Phenotype and metabolic characteristics of monocytes and granulocytes in preeclampsia. *Am J Obstet Gynecol*. 2001; **185**:792-95.

56. Chesley LC, Copper DW. Genetics of hypertension in pregnancy; Possible single gene control of pre-eclampsia and eclampsia in the descendents of eclamptic women. *Br J Obstet Gynecol* 1986; **93**:898-908.

57. Ners PB, Markovia N, Bars D. Family history of hypertension, heart disease and stroke among woman who developed hypertension. *Obstet Gynecol*. 2003; **102**:1366-69.

58. John JH, Ziebland S, Yudkin P. Effects of fruit and vegetable consumption on plasma antioxidant concentrations and blood pressure: A randomized controlled trail. *Lancet* 2002; **359**:1969-73.

59. Marcoux S, Brisson J, Fabia J. Calcium intake from dairy products and supplements and the risks of pre-eclampsia and gestational hypertension. *Am J Epidemiol* 1991; **133**:1266-72.

60. Juha R, William EW, Michael K, Leila R. Bone and Mineral metabolism. In Burtis CA, Ashwood ER, Bruns DE. Editors. Tietz text book of clinical chemistry and molecular diagnostics, Philadelphia: W.B Saunders 5th edn. 2012; 1733-1801.

61. Kovacs CS. Calcium and bone metabolism in pregnancy and lactation. *The Journal of Clinical Endocrinology and Metabolism* 2001; **86**:2344–2348.

62. Oliveri B, Parisi MS, Zeni S, Mautalen C. Mineral and bone mass changes during pregnancy and lactation. *Nutrition* 2004; **20**:235–240.

63. Atallah AN, Hofmeyr GJ, Duley L. Calcium supplementation during pregnancy for preventing hypertensive disorders and related problems. *The Cochrane Database of Systematic Reviews* 2004; **2**.

64. Patterson WB. Calcium deficiency as the prime cause of hypertension in pregnancy: A hypothesis. *Asia-Oceania Journal of Obstetrics and Gynecology* 1984; **10**:485–498.

65. Simpson KR, Creehan PA. Association of women's health, obstetric, and neonatal nurses. Perinatal nursing, Philadelphia: Lippincott 2nd edn. 2001.

66. Levine RJ, Hauth JC, Curet LB, Sibai BM, Catalano PM, Morris CD. Trial of calcium to prevent preeclampsia. *The New England Journal of Medicine* 1997; **337**:69–76.

67. Frolich A, Rudnicki M, Storm T, Rasmussen N, Hegedus L. Impaired 1,25- dihydroxy vitamin D production in pregnancy-induced hypertension. *Eur J Obstet Gynecol Reprod Biol* 1992; **47**:25-9.

68. Varner MW, Cruikshank JP, Pitkin RM. Calcium metabolism in hypertensive mother, fetus and new born infant. *Am J Obstet Gynecol* 1983; **147**:762-5.

69. Ritchie LD, King JC. Dietary calcium and pregnancy induced hypertension: is there a relation? *American Journal of Clinical Nutrition* 2000; **71**(5):1371S-1374S.

70. Myatt L. The relation of calcium nutrition and metabolism to pre-eclampsia and premature labour. In Tsang RC, Mimouni F, editors. Calcium nutrition for mothers and children. *New York: Raven Press*; 1992; 129-41.

71. Foley KF, Boccuzzi L. Urine Calcium: Laboratory Measurement and Clinical Utility. *Labmedicine* **41**(11) Nov 2010.

72. Fawcett WJ, Haxby EJ, Male DA. Magnesium: Physiology and Pharmacology. *Br J Anaesth* 1999; **83**:302-20.

73. Singh A, Verma AK, Hassan G, Prakash V, Sharma P, Kulshrestha S. Serum magnesium levels in patients with pre-eclampsia and eclampsia with different regimens of magnesium sulphate. *Global journal of medicine and public health* 2013; **2**(1).

74. Shear R, Leduc L, Rey E, Moutquin JM. Hypertension in pregnancy: New recommendations for management. *Curr. Hypert. Reports* 1999; 1:529-539.

75. Nadler JL, Goodson S, Rude RK. Evidence that prostacyclin mediates the vascular action of magnesium in humans. Hypertension 1987; **9**:379-383.

76. Cotton DB, Gonek B, Dorman KR. Cardiovascular alterations in severe pregnancy induced hypertension: acute effects of intravenous magnesium sulphate. *Am J Obstet. Gynecol.* 1984; **148**:162-165.

77. Scardo JA, Hogg BB, Newman RB. Favouralbe hemodynamic effects of magnesium sulphate in pre-eclampsia. *Am J Obstet. Gynecol* 1995; **173**:1249-1253.

78. Sipes S, Weiner C, Gellhaus T, Goodspeed J. Effect of magnesium sulphate infusion upon plasma prostaglandins in pre-eclampsia and preterm labour. *Hypertens pregnancy* 1994; **13**:293-302.

79. Lamb EJ and Price CP. Kidney Function Tests In: Burtis CA, Ashwood ER, Bruns DE. Editors. Tietz text book of clinical chemistry and molecular diagnostics 5th edn: Philadelphia: W.B Saunders 2012; 669-707.

80. Parks DA, Williams TK, Beckman JS. Conversion of xanthine dehydrogenase to oxidase in ischemic rat intestine: a reevaluation. *Am J Physiol.* 1988; **254**:G768–74.

81. Tan S, Gelman S, Wheat JK, Parks DA. Circulating xanthine oxidase in human ischemia reperfusion. *South Med J* 1995; **88**:479–82.

82. Lazzarino G, Raatikainen P, Nuutinen M, Nissinen J, Tavazzi B, Di Pierro D, Giardina B, Peuhkurinen K. Myocardial release of malondialdehyde and purine compounds during coronary bypass surgery. *Circulation* 1994; **90**:291-7.

83. White CR, Darley-Usmar V, Berrington WR, Mcadams M, Gore JZ, Thompson JA, Parks DA, Tarpey MM, Freeman BA. Circulating plasma xanthine oxidase contributes to vascular dysfunction in hypercholesterolemic rabbits. *Proc Natl Acad Sci U S A* 1996; **93**:8745-9.

84. Simic M and Jovanovic S. Antioxidation mechanisms of uric acid. J *Am Chem Soc.* 1989; **111**:5778-5782.

85. Johnson RJ, Kang DH, Feig D, Kivlighn S, Kanellis J, Watanabe S, Tuttle KR, Rodriguez-Iturbe B, Herrera-Acosta J, Mazzali M. Is there a pathogenetic role for uric acid in hypertension and cardiovascular and renal disease? Hypertension 2003; **41**:1183-90.

86. Galvan A, Natali A, Baldi S, Frascerra S, Sanna G, Ciociaro D, Ferrannini E. Effect of insulin on uric acid excretion in humans. *Am J Physiol.* 1995; **268**:E1-E5.

87. Carter J, Child A. Serum uric acid levels in normal pregnancy. *Aust N Z J Obstet Gynaecol.* 1989; **29**:313-4.

88. Powers RW, Bodnar LM, Ness RB, Cooper KM, Gallaher MJ, Frank MP, Daftary AR, Roberts JM. Uric acid concentrations in early pregnancy among preeclamptic women with gestational hyperuricemia at delivery. *Am J Obstet Gynecol.* 2006; **194**:160.

89. Voto LS, Illia R, Darbon-Grosso HA, Imaz FU, Margulies M. Uric acid levels: a useful index of the severity of preeclampsia and perinatal prognosis. *J Perinat Med.* 1988; **16**:123-6.

90. Roberts JM, Bodnar LM, Lain KY, Hubel CA, Markovic N, Ness RB, Powers RW. Uric acid is as important as proteinuria in identifying fetal risk in women with gestational hypertension. Hypertension 2005; **46**:1263-9.

91. Gallery ED, Hunyor SN, Gyory AZ. Plasma volume contraction: a significant factor in both pregnancy-associated hypertension (pre-eclampsia) and chronic hypertension in pregnancy. *Q J Med* 1979; **48**:593-602.

92. Bainbridge SA and Roberts JM. Uric Acid as a Pathogenic Factor in Preeclampsia. *Placenta* Mar 2008; **29**(Suppl A):S67–S72.

93. Pedersen EB, Johannesen P, Kristensen S, Ramussen AB, Emmertsen K, Moller J et al. Calcium, parathyroid hormone and calcitonin in normal pregnancy and pre-eclampsia. *Gynecol Obstet Invt.* 1984; **18**:156-63.

94. Taufield P, Ales KL, Resnick LM, Druzin ML, Gestnar JM, Laraugh JH. Hypocalciuria in pre-eclampsia. *N Eng J Med.* 1987; **316**:715-18.

95. Huikeshoven FJM and Zuiderhoudt FMJ. Hypocalciuria in hypertensive disorder of pregnancy and how to measure it. *Eur J Obstet Gynecol Reprod Biol.* 1990; **36**:81-85.

96. Vural P, Akgul C, Canbaz M. Calcium and Phosphate Excretion in Preeclampsia. *Turk J Med Sci* 2000; **30**:39–42.

97. Kazerooni T and Hamze-Nejadi S. Calcium to creatinine ratio in a spot sample of urine for early prediction of pre-eclampsia. *Int J Gynaecol Obstet.* Mar 2003; **80**(3):279-83.

98. Saudan PJ, Shaw L and Brown MA et al. Urinary calcium/creatinine ratio as a predictor of preeclampsia. *American Journal of Hypertension* Jul 1998; **11**(7):839-843.

99. Ozcan T, Kaleli B and Ozeren M et al. Urinary calcium to creatinine ratio for predicting preeclampsia. *Am J Perinatol.* Sep 1995; **12**(5):349-51.

100. Phuapradit W, Manusook S and Lolekha P. Urinary Calcium/Creatinine Ratio in the Prediction of Preeclampsia. *Australian and New Zealand Journal of Obstetrics and Gynaecology,* Aug 1993; **33**(3):280– 281.

101. Kazemi AFN, Sehhatie F, Sattarzade N and Mameghani ME. The Predictive Value of Urinary Calcium to Creatinine Ratio, Roll-Over Test and BMI in Early Diagnosis of Pre-Eclampsia. *Research Journal of Biological Sciences* 2010; **5**(2):183-186.

102. Ye Y, Dai S, Geng X. Predictive value of urinary calcium measurement on occurrence of pregnancy-induced hypertension. *Zhonghua Fu Chan Ke Za Zhi* Nov 1995; **30**(11):668-9.

103. Suzuki Y, Hayashi Y, Murakami I, Yamaguchi K, Yagami Y. Urinary calcium excretion as an early prediction marker for pregnancy induced hypertension. *Nihon Sanka Fujinka Gakkai Zasshi* Nov 1992; **44**(11):1421-6.

104. Kar J, Srivastava K, Mishra RK, Sharma N, Pandey ON, Gupta S. Role of urinary calcium creatinine ratio in prediction of pregnancy induced hypertension. *J Obstet Gynaecol. India* 2002; **52**(2):39-42.

105. Baker PN, Hackett GA. The use of urinary albumin–creatinine ratio and calcium–cratinine ratios as screening tests for pregnancy induced hypertension. *Obstet Gynaecol.* 1994; **83**:741-749.

106. Moni SY, Rashid MU, Begum HA, Ara S, Ahmed N. Role of Calcium Therapy on Urinary Calcium/Creatinine Ratio in healthy Pregnant Women and Pre-eclamptic Women. *Bangladesh J Physiol. Pharmacol.* 2009; **25**(1&2):7-9.

107. McGrowder D, Williams A, Gordon L, Crawford T, Alexander-Lindo R, Irving R, et al. Hypocalciuria in preeclampsia and gestational hypertension due to decreased fractional excretion of calcium. *Arch Med Sci.* 2009; **5**(1):80–85.

108. Raniolo E, Phillippou G. Prediction of PIH by means of urinary calcium creatinine ratio. *Med J Aus* 1993; **158**(2):98-100.

109. Kamra R, Gupta HP, Das K, Natu SM. Role of urinary calcium / creatinine ratio in the prediction of pregnancy induced hypertension. *J Obstet Gynecol India.* 1994; **47**(4):353-358.

110. Kisters K, Korner J, Louwen F, Witteler R, Jackisch C, Zidek W, Ott S, Westermann G, M Barenbrock, K H Rahn. Plasma and membrane Ca2+ and Mg2+ concentrations in normal pregnancy and in preeclampsia. *Gynecol Obstet Invest.* 1998; **46**(3):158-63.

111. Alavi A, Jahanshahi KA, Karimia S, Arabzadea N, Fallahi S. Comparison of serum calcium, total protein and uric acid levels between hypertensive and healthy pregnant women in an Iranian population. *Life Science Journal* 2012; **9**(4).

112. Kosch M, Hausberg M, Louwen F, Barenbrock M, Rahn KH, Kisters K. Alterations of plasma calcium and intracellular and membrane calcium in erythrocytes of patients with pre-eclampsia. *J Hum Hypertens.* May 2000; **14**(5):333-6.

113. Malas NO, Shurideh ZM. Does serum calcium in pre-eclampsia and normal pregnancy differ? *Saudi Med J.* Oct 2001; **22**(10):868-71.

114. Cunha AR, Umbelino B, Correia ML and Neves MF. Magnesium and Vascular Changes in Hypertension. *International Journal of Hypertension* 2012; Article ID 754250.

115. Touyz RM. Role of magnesium in the pathogenesis of hypertension. *Mol Aspects Med.* Feb-Jun 2003; **24**(1-3):107-36.

116. Seydoux J, Girardin E, Paunier L, Beguin F. Serum and intracellular magnesium during normal pregnancy and in patients with pre-eclampsia. *Br J Obstet Gynaecol.* Mar 1992; **99**(3):207-11.

117. Sayyed AK, Sonttake AN. Electrolyte Status in Preeclampsia. *Online International Interdisciplinary Research Journal* May-June 2013; **3**(3).4

118. Sendhav S, Khubchandani A, Gandhi P, Sanghani H, Sidhu G, Vadhel A. A Comparative Study of Serum Uric Acid, Calcium and Magnesium in Preeclampsia and Normal Pregnancy. *Journal of Advance Researches in Biological Sciences* 2013; **5**(1):55-58.

119. Weerasekera D S and Peiris H. The Significance of Serum Uric Acid, Creatinine and Urinary Microprotein levels in predicting Pre-Eclampsia. *Journal of and Obstetrics Gynaecology* 2003; 23(1):17-19. Thangaratinam S, Ismail KMK, Sharp S, Coomarasamy A, Khan KS. Accuracy of serum uric acid in predicting complications of pre-eclampsia: a systematic review. *An International Journal of Obstetrics and Gynaecology* Apr 2006; **113**(4):369-78.

120. Kang DH, Finch J, Nakagawa T, Karumanchi SA, Kanellis J, Granger J, Johnson RJ. Uric acid, endothelial dysfunction and pre-eclampsia: searching for a pathogenetic link. *J Hypertens.* Feb 2004; **22**(2):229-35.

121. Lam C, Lim KH, Kang DH, Karumanchi SA. Uric acid and preeclampsia. *Semin Nephrol.* Jan 2005; **25**(1):56-60.

122. Sahijwani D, Desai A, Oza H, Kansara V, Ninama P, Maheshwari K, Soni C. Serum Uric Acid as a Prognostic Marker of Pregnancy Induced Hypertension. *Journal of South Asian Federation of Obstetrics and Gynaecology*, Sep-Dec 2012; **4**(3):130-133.

123. Gaugler–Senden IPM, Roes EM, De-Groot CJM, Steegers EAP. Clinical risk factors for pre-eclampsia. *Eur Clinics Obstet Gynaecol* 2005; **1**:36-50.

124. Dutta DC, Konar H. Textbook of Obstetrics. New Central Book Agency (P) Ltd. 6th Edn. 2004; 222-223.

125. Gibbs RS, Karlan BY, Hanney AF, Nygaard I. Danforth's text book of Obstetrics and Gynecology. Lippincott Williams and Wilkins 10th Edn. 2008; 259.

126. Izumi A, Minakami H, Kuwata T et al. Calcium to creatinine ratio in spot urine samples in early pregnancy and its relation to the development of preeclampsia. Metabolism 1997; **46**:107-8.

128. Frenkel Y, Barkai G, Mashiach S, Dolev E, Zimlichman R, Weiss M. Hypocalciuria of preeclampsia is independent of parathyroid hormone level. *Obstet* 1991; **77**:689–691.

129. Szmidt-Adjide V, Vendittelli F, David S, Bredent-Bangou J, Janky E. Calciuria and preeclampsia: a case-control study. *Eur J Obstet Gynecol Reprod Biol.* 2006; **125**(2):193–198.

130. Mandira D, Sudhir A, Mamtaz S. Urinary calcium levels in preeclampsia. *J Obstet Gynecol India* 2008; **58**(4):308–311.

131. Gasnier RGEG, Vettorazzi J, Martins-Costa SH, Barros EG, Ramos JGL. Calcium to creatinine ratio in pregnancy-induced hypertension. *International Society for the Study of Hypertension in Pregnancy* 2011; S2210-7789(11)00239-X.

132. Almasganj F, Asghari L, Shokohi H. Study of relation between calcium and uric acid level with hypertensive disorder in pregnancy and result of pregnancy. *Journal of Medical Council of Islamic Republic of Iran* 2004; **22**(1):10-14.

133. Taner C, Guler A, Basogul O, Nayaki UA, Ersoy GY, Derin G. Serum uric acid measurements in hypertensive disorders of pregnancy. *T Klin J Gynecol Obst* 2004; **14**:32-36.